THE STATE OF THE WORLD'S CHILDREN
1994

SERVICES

Oxford University Press, Walton Street,
Oxford, OX2 6DP, Oxfordshire, U.K.
Oxford, New York, Toronto, Delhi, Bombay,
Calcutta, Madras, Karachi, Peealing Jaya,
Singapore, Hong Kong, Tokyo, Nairobi,
Dar-es-Salaam, Cape Town, Melbourne,
Auckland and associated companies in
Beirut, Berlin, Ibadan, Nicosia.

Oxford is a trade mark of Oxford University
Press.
Published in the United States by
Oxford University Press, New York.

Any part of The State of the World's Children
may be freely reproduced with the
appropriate acknowledgement.

British Library Cataloguing in
Publication Data
The state of the world's children 1994
1. Children – Care and hygiene
613' 0432 RJ101
ISBN 0-19-262484-9

ISSN 0265-718X

The Library of Congress has catalogued this
serial publication as follows:-
The state of the world's children – Oxford and
New York: Oxford University Press for UNICEF
v.; ill.; 20cm. Annual. Began publication in
1980.
1. Children -Developing countries - Periodicals.
2. Children - Care and hygiene - eveloping
countries - Periodicals. I. UNICEF.
HQ 792.2.S73 83-647550 362.7' 1'091724

UNICEF, UNICEF House, 3 U.N. Plaza,
New York, N.Y. 10017, U.S.A.
UNICEF, Palais des Nations, CH. 1211
Geneva 10, Switzerland.

Design: Threefold, Witney, U.K.
Charts: Stephen Hawkins, Oxford, U.K.
Cover photo: Peter Williams/W.C.C.
Printing: Burgess (Abingdon) Ltd., U.K.

Edited and produced for UNICEF and
Oxford University Press by P & L Adamson,
18 Observatory Close, Benson, Wallingford,
Oxon OX10 6NU, U.K.
tel 0491-838431, fax 0491-825426

THE STATE
OF THE WORLD'S
CHILDREN
1994

James P. Grant
Executive Director of the
United Nations Children's Fund
(UNICEF)

PUBLISHED FOR UNICEF

Oxford University Press

Contents

Text figures

Panels

"The necessary task of drawing attention to human needs has unfortunately given rise to the popular impression that the developing world is a stage upon which no light falls and only tragedy is enacted. But the fact is that, for all the set-backs, more progress has been made in the last 50 years than in the previous 2,000. Since the end of the Second World War, average real incomes in the developing world have more than doubled; infant and child death rates have been more than halved; average life expectancy has increased by about a third; the proportion of the developing world's children starting school has risen to more than three quarters; and the percentage of rural families with access to safe water has increased from less than 10% to almost 60%.

"Over that same time, much of the world has also freed itself from colonialism, brought apartheid in all its forms to the edge of extinction, and largely freed itself from the iron grip of fascist and totalitarian regimes.

"In the decade ahead, a clear opportunity exists to make the breakthrough against what might be called the last great obscenity - the needless malnutrition, disease, and illiteracy that still cast a shadow over the lives, and the futures, of the poorest quarter of the world's children."

The State of the World's Children 1993

Introduction and summary of themes

Through the lens of history, rather than of news, what is now happening in the developing world may come to be seen as the beginning of a final offensive against some of the oldest and most common enemies of the world's children.

Those enemies include five diseases that today kill over 8 million children a year and the malnutrition which holds back the mental and physical development of one child in three in the developing world (fig. 1). Also in retreat are some of the most common causes of childhood disability, the viruses and the micronutrient deficiencies which every year leave hundreds of thousands of children permanently deaf, blind, mentally retarded, or paralysed.

Although profoundly affecting millions of lives, these tragedies, and the progress now being made against them, are largely neglected by the media. In part, this is because these problems are seen as normal rather than exceptional. But primarily it is because their consequences fall almost exclusively on the children of the poorest and least influential people on earth.

The limited good news of recent years is therefore largely an untold story in the midst of the many well-publicized disasters. Measles, for example, which still kills more children every year than all the world's wars and famines put together, is being forced to relinquish its grip. Deaths from this most devastating of childhood diseases

have been brought down from more than 2.5 million a year in 1980 to just over 1 million a year today. Simultaneously, the number of non-fatal cases of measles, a major cause of disability and malnutrition in children, has fallen from approximately 75 million a year to about 25 million.

Similar successes have been recorded, by dint of large-scale but little-recognized efforts in the developing world, against several other major problems facing the children of poor communities. In 10 years, infant deaths from neonatal tetanus have been cut from more than 1 million a year to just over half a million. At the same time, the toll of dehydration caused by diarrhoeal disease has been cut from 4 million deaths a year to less than 3 million.

Polio, which has disabled so many millions of children over the years, is also now in retreat. Since 1980, new cases of paralysis have fallen from approximately half a million a year to an estimated 140,000 in 1992. In several regions of the developing world the virus itself is close to being eradicated. As an overall measure of this achievement, it is now estimated that there are more than 3 million children living normal lives who would have been paralysed by polio had it not been for the increase in immunization coverage in the last decade.

At the end of the 1980s, the internationally agreed target of 80% immunization against the major vaccine-preventable diseases of childhood was

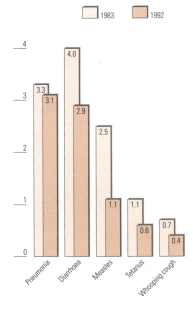

Fig. 1 Major diseases

Under-five deaths from major diseases of childhood in the developing world (millions).

The above reductions in deaths from particular diseases have been achieved despite an increase of approximately 20% in the number of under-fives (1983-1992).

WHO estimates for the annual number of measles deaths have been recently revised. The figure given here may not tally with previous years' reports.

1983 figures do not include China.

Source: *World Health Organization, 1993.*

reached by almost half of the developing countries. Nearly all reached a coverage level of 70% or more (fig. 2). By 1995, there is a reasonable chance that several other internationally agreed goals will also have been largely achieved.

Iodine deficiency, which causes 120,000 children a year to be born as cretins and is the world's major cause of preventable mental retardation, could soon be brought to an end.

Vitamin A deficiency, which blinds an estimated 250,000 children a year and is a major cause of ill health and early death among the world's under-fives, could be almost eliminated.

Deaths from neonatal tetanus, preventable by the immunization of pregnant women, should soon become a rarity.

Proper treatment of diarrhoeal disease, including oral rehydration therapy (ORT), should be known to 80% of the developing world's families: the result would be the prevention of a further 1.5 million child deaths each year.

Polio should be eradicated from most countries of the world by 1995.

Meanwhile, progress is also being made towards the universal ratification of the Convention on the Rights of the Child, now ratified by 150 nations of which 28 have so far reported on the steps they have taken towards its full implementation.

The bad news, though more widely travelled, cannot be ignored. Problems of the most acute kind – extremes of deprivation and exploitation, and the inhuman abuse of children in war, in the workplace, on the street, and in the home – continue to afflict many millions of young people in both developing and industrialized countries. But even here, there are the first tentative signs of a new ethic emerging which might one day offer children better protection from the worst evils of the adult world. This fragile hope is discussed in panel 1.

The PPE spiral

In keeping with its tradition of focusing on changes which touch the lives of large numbers of children but which rarely make headlines, part 1 of this year's *State of the World's Children* report summarizes the progress being made against the major specific threats to the health and nutrition of children in the world's poorest communities. It also outlines the potential for further significant advances in the years immediately ahead.

Part 2 sets this progress and potential in the context of the broader problems that cloud humanity's prospects in the 21st century. In particular, it looks at the mutually reinforcing relationships between the worst effects of absolute poverty, the continuation of rapid population growth, and the degradation of rural and urban environments throughout much of the developing world. So interrelated have these problems become that to denominate them separately is to risk misconstruing the threat that they represent; for this reason, the report unites the issues of poverty, population growth, and environment under the term 'the PPE problem'.

The PPE problem is itself part of an even broader challenge. For it is becoming clear that the world has only a limited time in which to focus its attention and capacities on managing what will undoubtedly be the most complex and difficult transition in all of human history – the transition to a new path of progress characterized by the universal meeting of minimum human needs, by the stabilization and possible reduction of population levels, and by environmentally sustainable patterns of progress in all nations. It is also evident that this multifaceted challenge will demand all of the technological ingenuity, managerial capacity, and political acuity that national societies and the international community can command. Negotiating this great transition must therefore replace the military and ideological preoccupations of the past, and become the new central organizing principle of the post-cold war world.

Although this report centres on the PPE problem in the developing world, it should be made clear at the outset

Negotiating the transition to a sustainable future must become the central organizing principle of the post-cold war era.

that the transition to a sustainable future is largely the responsibility of the established industrialized countries. The path pioneered by a small group of nations over the last five centuries has brought to the rest of the world many benefits amid much pain. It has also pushed the tolerance of the biosphere close to breaking-point. Overwhelmingly, global environmental pressures arise from the already industrialized nations. Such a state of affairs cannot long continue, both because the industrialized world's levels of consumption and pollution are in themselves unjust and unsustainable, and because the other four fifths of the world cannot reasonably be expected to restrain or modify the course of its own development in order to protect the biosphere while the industrialized nations continue to monopolize the earth's capacity to provide and to absorb.

This challenge, which many are unwilling to think about today, will become more and more unavoidable as the 21st century begins.

For the industrialized world, the most difficult challenge will undoubtedly be the redefining of its own concepts of growth and progress. But if the great transition is to be made, then it is clear that the industrialized nations will also have to play a major part in resolving the PPE problem in the developing world.

In the face of all the immediate political and economic issues that command the attention of press, public, and politicians in all countries, it might be expected that the problems faced by the poorest people in the poorest countries would continue to occupy a lowly place on the international agenda. But sooner or later this too will have to change. For it will simply not be possible to negotiate the transitions that lie ahead without addressing the PPE problem in the poorest communities of the world. Within a very few years, failure to cope with the combined impact of the worst aspects of poverty, rapid population growth, and environmental decline will almost certainly translate itself into increasing social division,

economic disruption, political unrest, and the gradual dwindling of the present opportunity for progress towards democracy and international stability. From the consequences of such a failure, no country – north or south, rich or poor – would be immune.

Action now

Part 3 of the report unites the themes of progress for today's children with the longer-term PPE problem. Its central argument is that pursuing today's low-cost opportunities to protect the health, nutrition, and education of women and children in the developing world is one of the most immediately available and affordable ways of weakening the grip of poverty, population growth, and environmental deterioration.

In particular, it seeks to show that the PPE problem will not be resolved without a sustained national and international effort to overcome the very worst aspects of poverty in the remaining years of this century. For poverty is the root of the population and environment crisis in the developing world, and it is also the most accessible point at which to break into the powerful synergisms which form the downward spiral of PPE problems.

What is now required is a determined effort to protect millions of children from the very worst effects of the poverty into which they are born. Today's knowledge and outreach capacity make it possible, for the first time, to protect the mental and physical development of almost all the world's children. It has therefore become possible to interrupt one of the major processes by which poverty is perpetuated from one generation to the next.

An adequate response to the PPE problem must therefore include, among many other actions in many other fields, at least four basic kinds of investment in the lives of the world's poorest communities. They are:

☐ The prevention of common diseases and disabilities, and a steep reduction in both severe and moderate malnutrition;

☐ Rapid progress towards at least a

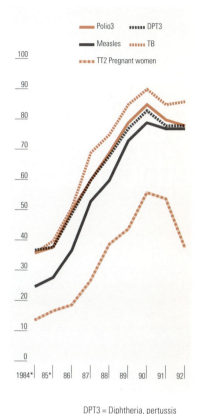

Fig. 2 Immunization coverage

Percentage of the developing world's one-year-olds protected against the major vaccine-preventable diseases.

DPT3 = Diphtheria, pertussis (whooping cough), and tetanus vaccine (3 doses).

TT2 = Tetanus toxoid vaccine for pregnant women (2 doses).

*Excluding China.

Source: *WHO and UNICEF, August 1993.*

3

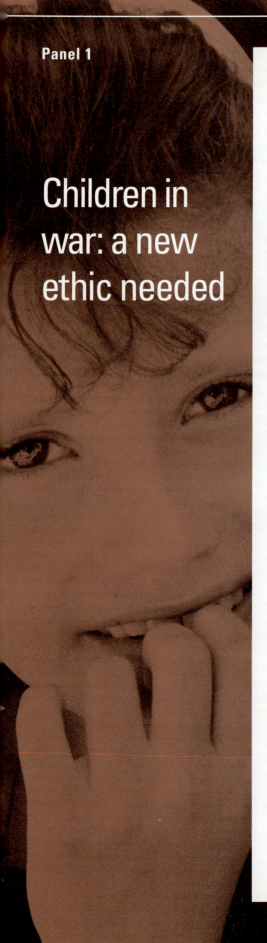

Children in war: a new ethic needed

In the 1990s, the world stands at a critical juncture for the cause of protecting children in war.

On the one hand, it appears that an alarming retrogression is occurring. In previous eras, the main casualties of wars have been soldiers. No longer. In the last decade alone, an estimated 1.5 million children have been killed in armed conflicts. A further 4 million have been disabled, maimed, blinded, brain-damaged. At least 5 million have become refugees, and 12 million more have been uprooted from their communities. Much larger numbers have seen their health, nutrition, and education suffer as conflicts have destroyed crops, infrastructure, clinics, schools.

More recently, the rape of girls has been used as a systematic weapon of war in former Yugoslavia. And in many parts of the world, children have been tortured and forced to watch or participate in atrocities. Hundreds of thousands have been crippled by land-mines. Many more have been recruited into armies, given drugs and weapons, and desensitized to others' pain. Uncounted millions of these young people are suffering from post-traumatic stress disorders, a new and chilling term in the international lexicon.

In the face of an unprecedented number of such reports, it seems right to conclude that the veneer of civilization has never before been worn so thin.

At the same time, there are also some signs of a new commitment to protect children from the worst evils of the adult world. The intense media reporting of atrocities concerning children is itself an example, as is the worldwide public response and the rapid rise in the number of dedicated non-governmental organizations, in all countries, who are working to prevent the abuse of children in war and to offer help to those already victimized.

The Declaration signed by the world's political leaders at the 1990 World Summit for Children specifically asked "*that periods of tranquillity and special relief corridors be observed for the benefit of children, where war and violence are still taking place*". Also in the 1990s, a new framework for all such efforts has emerged in the shape of the Convention on the Rights of the Child, which incorporates specific provisions for the protection of children in armed conflicts as well as proclaiming the right of all children to basic health care, nutrition, and education. In its first four years, the Convention has been ratified by some 150 Governments. No other human rights convention has ever progressed to this first stage so rapidly. It is UNICEF's hope that by 1995 the Convention will have been ratified by all 184 members of the United Nations – setting a standard for the survival, protection, and development of children below which any nation should be ashamed to fall.

In recent years, this emerging movement has begun to achieve practical results. Beginning with 'the days of tranquillity' which allowed El Salvador's children to be immunized on several days of each year during that nation's civil war, the notion has been gaining ground that protection for children should be agreed to by all parties in time of war. National immunization days in Lebanon, and 'corridors of peace' during the fighting in the Sudan, are other examples of this embryonic principle going into action, as are the efforts to meet the essential needs of children at the height of the Gulf War and in Sarajevo's darkest days.

As with all such principles, advance in the real world has been by means of two steps forward and one back. And progress can only be maintained by a loud and insistent public demand for action. □

primary education for all children, and especially for all girls;

☐ An unprecedented worldwide effort to improve the lives of women in poor communities – their health and education, their status and choices, their rights and opportunities. This is an important issue of principle; it is also the most important practical step that could be taken towards weakening the hold of the PPE problem;

☐ The making available of family planning information and services to all who need them.

In sum, the central message of this year's report is that making further investments in the well-being of women and children – investments which are at risk of being neglected in the face of newer and seemingly more dramatic problems – is not only one of the most important humanitarian goals that the world could set for itself, but also one of the most incisive and cost-effective contributions that could be made towards coping with the broader problems of poverty, population growth, and environmental deterioration.

The cost of making such an investment in the 1990s would amount to not much more than one tenth of 1% of the world's annual economic product.

It is a rare bargain. And one that the world cannot afford to miss.

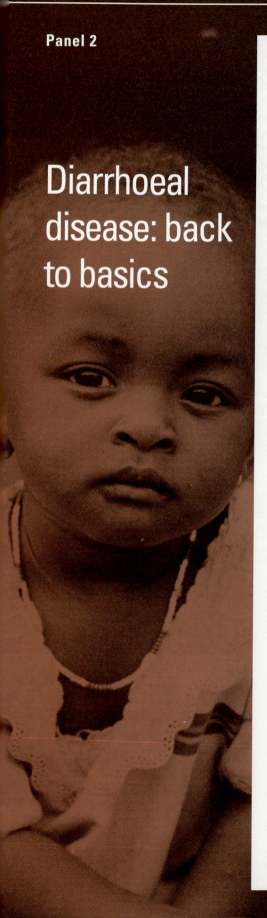

Diarrhoeal disease: back to basics

A quarter-century after it was introduced to the world, oral rehydration therapy (ORT) is now saving over 1 million young lives a year.

ORT means increased fluid intake and continued feeding when a child has diarrhoea. It is low-cost and doable at home, with or without packets of prepared oral rehydration salts (ORS). And it has proved the best safeguard against the often deadly dehydration that drains away the body's vital fluids. It is also now the standard procedure taught at some of the world's most prestigious medical schools.

Few in medical or government circles, schools or families knew about ORT when UNICEF moved the formula to the top of its agenda, along with immunization, at the start of the 1980s. Today, one in three children stricken with diarrhoea receives ORT at home. The result is the prevention of about 3,000 child deaths each day. ORT should always include continued feeding – and can also help to keep malnutrition at bay for even larger numbers of children.

Far too often, however, ORT is ignored. More than 2 million under-fives in the world's poorest neighbourhoods still die needlessly every year of diarrhoeal dehydration. And it remains a primary cause of malnutrition: recurrent diarrhoea robs a child's body of nutrients, reduces appetite and inhibits food absorption.

To accelerate progress, the leaders of most developing countries, with the encouragement of WHO and UNICEF, have set the goal of 80% ORT use by the end of 1995.

But the example of Egypt shows the importance of sustaining efforts over the long term. In 1983, the Government, backed by the United States Agency for International Development, launched a highly successful ORS promotion campaign. Within two years, 96% of mothers with young children had heard about oral rehydration, and the ORS usage rate surpassed 50%. Partly as a result, under-five mortality dropped by nearly half, from 136 to 72 per 1,000 between 1985 and 1991.

Yet external funding for Egypt's ORS programme has waned, and current ORT usage rates are down to 34%. A major stumbling-block is the medical profession; it has proved very difficult to convince doctors, especially doctors in private practice, that so simple an approach should be the first-choice treatment. Drug therapy remains the preferred route: recent surveys by WHO of two Egyptian governorates showed ORS was used in 23% of cases of diarrhoeal disease, while drugs were prescribed in 54%.

Only one in ten diarrhoea cases requires antibiotics as well as oral rehydration. ORS sachets, widely available at no more than 10 cents each, and home remedies such as rice water, weak tea or green coconut water, can forestall most dehydration. Yet drug treatment overwhelms ORS use in most countries. According to WHO, more than $1 billion is spent each year, in developing and developed countries alike, on useless and often harmful antidiarrhoeal medicines.

Some countries are returning to basics. Under the direct personal supervision of President Carlos Salinas, Mexico has just launched a two-year $20 million drive to bring oral rehydration to every child in every state. Under the banner 'The best solution', the campaign stresses the 'three Fs' – fluids, food, and further help when a child requires a doctor. To back up the publicity, national women's organizations are training neighbourhood mothers, whose homes then fly the white flag of the campaign; and correct case management is being taught to medical personnel across the nation – in hospitals and private practice as well as in the new oral rehydration centres. □

A progress report

The most important aspect of the progress now being achieved for children in the developing world is the gradual ascendancy that is being gained over the major diseases of childhood.

The most devastating of those diseases is common measles, a relatively minor illness in the industrialized nations but a major cause of death, malnutrition, and disability among the children of poor communities in the developing world.* Not much more than a decade ago, approximately 75 million children contracted the measles virus each year, and more than 2.5 million died during the acute phase of the illness. Today, thanks to improvements in health care and immunization, measles cases have been reduced to approximately 25 million a year and deaths from the disease have been cut to just over 1 million.[1]

Second, significant progress is also being made against the diarrhoeal diseases that are among the major causes of stunted growth and early death among the children of poor communities. In the early 1980s, approximately 4 million children a year were dying from diarrhoeal disease. But since 1985, the technique of ORT has been put at the disposal of approximately 250 million families or about one third of the developing world's children. Sixty countries now produce packets of oral rehydration salts (ORS) to the formula developed by the World Health Organization (WHO) and UNICEF, and more than two thirds of the world's population can obtain ORS within a reasonable distance from their homes.[2] The result is the prevention of more than 1 million deaths a year from diarrhoeal disease (panel 2).[3]

The 1980s and early 1990s have also seen the raising of immunization levels from under 20% to approximately 80% – undoubtedly one of the greatest public health achievements of this or any other century. In addition to its contribution to measles control, immunization has also made major inroads into territories formerly held by whooping cough, tetanus, diphtheria, and polio. At the beginning of the 1980s, whooping cough was killing over 700,000 children a year; today that toll has been reduced to approximately 400,000.[4] Over the same period, the number of newborns dying from neonatal tetanus has fallen from 1.1 million to less than 600,000 (panel 3) and the number of children dying from diphtheria has been cut from 19,000 to 4,000.[5]

Also as a result of immunization efforts, polio has been steadily giving ground. In 1980, almost 400,000 children were crippled for life by the polio virus. Last year, its victims numbered approximately 140,000 (panel 4 and fig. 3).[6] According to WHO, there is now a reasonable chance that polio can be eradicated from the face of the earth by the year 2000.

A lesser-known benefit of progress in immunization is its contribution to improved nutrition. Frequent illnesses are a threat to a child's nutritional health and long-term growth: they reduce appetite for several days at a time; they inhibit the absorption of food; they consume calories in fevers and in fighting the disease; and they drain away nutrients in vomiting and diarrhoea. When such illnesses strike frequently, the child is steadily pushed into a downward spiral of malnutrition and ill health. And it is this spiral, rather than any individual cause, which results in so many millions of children failing to survive their early years or failing to grow to their full mental and physical potential (panel 5). The major gains being made against specific childhood diseases in recent years therefore also represent a significant gain against the fundamental problems

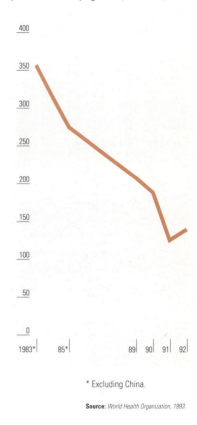

Fig. 3 Polio cases

Estimated annual number of children contracting polio in the developing world (thousands).

* Excluding China.

Source: *World Health Organization, 1993.*

* Nearly 2 million young lives are therefore being saved each year by the control of measles. But the significance of this achievement goes considerably beyond the prevention of death: it is increasingly recognized that non-fatal attacks of measles are strongly associated with malnutrition, pneumonia, diarrhoea, vitamin A loss, encephalitis, conjunctivitis, otitis media, blindness, and deafness. The prevention of 50 million cases of this disease each year therefore represents a major improvement in the general health and nutrition of the developing world's children.

Fig. 4 Fertility falls

Total fertility rate (average number of births per woman) since 1960.

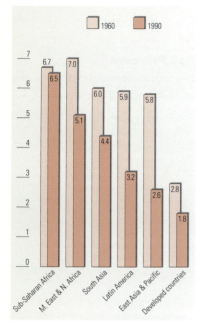

The total fertility rate is the number of children that would be born to a woman who lives to the end of her child-bearing years and who bears children at each age in accordance with prevailing age-specific fertility rates.

Source: *United Nations*, World population prospects: the 1992 revision, *1993*.

of malnutrition and poor mental and physical development. In other words, they are significant steps towards eradicating not only symptoms but causes of poverty and underdevelopment.

Recent years have also seen steady progress in extending safe water and sanitation to millions of families in the developing world. Since 1980, the proportion of families with access to safe drinking water has risen from 38% to 68% in South-East Asia, from 66% to 78% in Latin America, and from 32% to 43% in Africa.[7] Safe sanitation has advanced more slowly, but more than half of all families in the developing world can now dispose of faeces safely.[8] These gains too have made their contribution to reducing the toll of disease and improving nutritional health.

Lastly, remarkable progress has also been made in extending the knowledge and the means of family planning. In three decades, the number of children born to the average woman in the developing world has fallen from 6.0 to 3.7 (fig. 4). Overall, the proportion of married women using modern methods of family planning has increased from less than 10% to approximately 50% (fig. 5).[9] The speed of this change is unprecedented in demographic history, with some 17 nations succeeding in halving their fertility rates in only one generation.[10] *"The most significant development in reproductive health over the past few decades,"* says Dr. Hiroshi Nakajima, Director-General of WHO, *"has been the major expansion in the use of contraceptives, with major benefits to individuals, families, societies, and the world at large."*[11]

As part 3 of this report will show, family planning is one of the most important of all contributions to social and economic development: it reduces the number of maternal deaths; it lowers under-five mortality rates; it improves the nutritional health of both women and children; it gives women more health, more time, and more opportunity; it has a positive impact on the care and education of children; and it slows population growth. And even though there is still a considerable unmet demand, the spread of family

planning constitutes one of the most significant contributions to human well-being of recent years.

Social change

Advances in knowledge and technology have been necessary but not sufficient to bring about these improvements. Most of the science involved has, after all, been available for several decades: ORT proved its large-scale effectiveness 25 years ago;[12] the vaccines that have made possible recent progress against measles, tetanus, whooping cough, and polio have been available since at least the 1960s; most of the modern methods of contraception now in widespread use have been available for 30 years; and salt iodization was first used to overcome iodine deficiency disorders in Switzerland and the United States during the 1920s.

The new element which has made possible the recent mass application of these advances is a wider social and economic change. Linked to gradual economic growth, that social change has been of two main kinds. First, infrastructure and communications capacity in most developing nations have now reached the point at which it is physically and financially possible to bring the basic benefits of scientific progress to virtually every community. This is a historic and much underestimated change, and its potential has been forcefully demonstrated by the immunization achievements of recent years. High levels of immunization coverage in the developing world indicate that a system is now in place – including a capacity for training, supply, management, communications, delivery, and record-keeping – that is capable of reaching out to over 100 million infants a year on four or five separate occasions during their first year of life. That outreach system, extending to almost every rural hamlet and urban neighbourhood, is very far from being universally reliable, and it will require extraordinary efforts to sustain and strengthen it in the remaining years of the 1990s; but its achievements so far have shown that almost all developing nations now have the capacity to put the basic benefits of scientific progress at the disposal of almost all of their people.

The second and related change is the rise in worldwide public and political awareness that such advances are now possible, that both the scientific knowledge and the outreach capacity are now available, and that it is simply no longer necessary, and therefore no longer acceptable, for millions of families to endure preventable disease and malnutrition and for millions of their children to suffer frequent illness, poor growth, and early death. *"Today, the world is both aware that this tragedy is happening and capable of preventing it,"* said the *State of the World's Children* report for 1989. *"Ethics must march with awareness, morality with capacity."*

This message of what it is now possible to achieve has arisen from health practitioners and schools of public health, from United Nations agencies, from the foundations and the non-governmental organizations, from the professional bodies and the research institutions, and from increasing numbers of activists, media commentators, opinion leaders, and political bodies.

As that voice has grown in volume, so it has begun to translate itself into political pressures. An early example was the commitment to the 80% immunization goal made by almost all national political leaders in the mid-1980s. At that time, only a third of the developing world's children were being immunized: just over five years later, close to 80% were being protected by vaccines.

At about the same time as the immunization goal was being reached, this process of widening awareness and growing pressure for action was leading to specific demands for other basic benefits of progress to be made universally available. To thousands of individuals and organizations all over the world, it began to seem more and more of an outrage that something as simple, preventable, and treatable as ordinary diarrhoeal disease was still claiming the lives of 3 million young children a year; or that more than 3 million were being allowed to die from respiratory infections when antibiotics could be made available at almost negligible cost; or that the world was still prepared to tolerate millions of deaths a year from measles, whooping cough, and tetanus among the 20% of children who were still not being reached by vaccines; or that poliomyelitis was still being allowed to paralyse more than 100,000 children a year when it had become possible to eradicate the virus from the face of the earth.

As the 1980s progressed, a rapid expansion in knowledge about the condition of children in developing countries began to add other issues to this list. Why were a quarter of a million children a year being allowed to go blind from the lack of vitamin A when it was possible to make inexpensive vitamin A capsules available to every child at risk?[13] Why was iodine deficiency still the leading cause of preventable mental retardation in the world (fig. 6), causing over 100,000 infants to be born as cretins each year and affecting the normal development of at least 50 million children, when the problem could be prevented by something as affordable and manageable as iodizing all salt supplies?[14] Why were an estimated 1 million babies being allowed to die each year because of an almost unchallenged decline in the practice of exclusive breastfeeding in many areas of the world?[15] And why were nearly a million people still suffering the painful and debilitating effects of guinea worm disease when the cost of control in affected areas had been reduced to only about $2.50 per person?[16]

Even areas in which steady progress had been made began to be subjected to a more impatient questioning. Why do a billion people still lack safe water when new technologies and community-based strategies (panel 6) have shown the way to solve this problem at much reduced cost?[17] Why are a third of the developing world's children below an acceptable weight when new approaches have demonstrated that malnutrition can be very substantially reduced at a cost of less than $10 per child?[18] Why do sur-

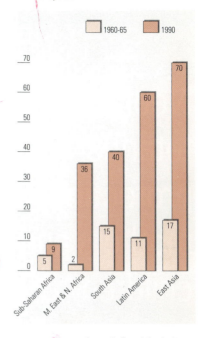

Fig. 5 Family planning

Percentage of married women using some form of contraception.

1960-65   1990

Source: *John Ross and others,* Family planning and child survival programs as assessed in 1991, *Population Council, 1992.*

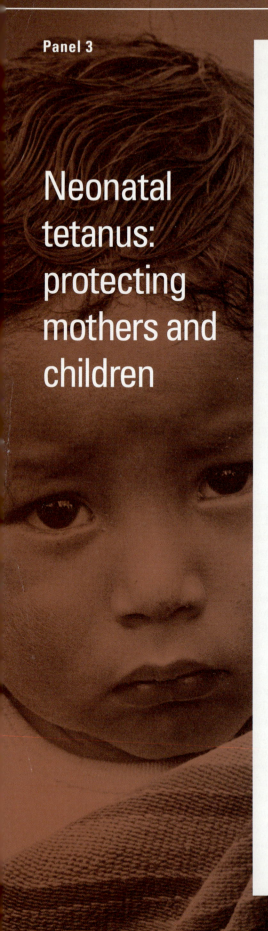

Neonatal tetanus: protecting mothers and children

Every minute, a newborn dies of tetanus infection. Every ten minutes, the same disease strikes down a new mother. Every year, an estimated 50,000 maternal deaths and nearly 600,000 neonatal tetanus deaths – or up to one quarter of infant mortality in some countries – could be prevented by tetanus vaccination and clean birth practices.

One of the goals adopted by the 1990 World Summit for Children was the elimination of neonatal tetanus by 1995. The vaccine itself has been available for 30 years, and it has long been known that two doses of tetanus toxoid during pregnancy will protect both mother and baby until the child can be vaccinated independently.

Yet the effort to defeat tetanus lags badly behind. After a decade of intense effort, the immunization of infants against other vaccine-preventable diseases reached or neared 80% in most countries by the end of 1990. Coverage of pregnant women with tetanus vaccine rose from under 15% to about 55% over the decade, but has since fallen back to less than 40%.

Four years ago, the *State of the World's Children* report cited the comment of Dr. Ralph Henderson, who directed the World Health Organization's Expanded Programme on Immunization for most of the 1980s:

"*The continuance of neonatal tetanus represents a major failure of public health practice. It is one of the most dramatic and angering indications of our wider failure to provide basic maternal health services. Not one case of neonatal tetanus should be allowed to occur. Before 1995, the disease should be eliminated in every country. We have a good, stable vaccine and it could and should have been done yesterday.*"

Sadly, those words are just as relevant today.

The 'wider failure' includes the unsafe birth practices which bring tetanus spores into contact with the unhealed umbilical cord or birth canal. Large numbers of women in the developing world give birth in circumstances of poor hygiene and medical neglect. According to the World Health Organization, only half of all deliveries are considered 'clean' and only half are attended by a trained person.

Some countries are winning the battle against tetanus by a combination of vaccinations and efforts to promote safer childbirth. Zimbabwe, where three out of five pregnant women are fully immunized against tetanus, now trains all women who perform deliveries, with an emphasis on the 'three cleans' – clean hands, a clean surface for delivery, and clean cutting and care of the cord. And China, where the idea of the three cleans was first developed, recently began its first tetanus vaccination campaign for women in 300 counties.

Thailand, where tetanus used to cause one quarter of neonatal mortality, is on the way to wiping out the disease by 1995. The campaign stresses improved reporting of cases, mass education to motivate women to be vaccinated, and teaching safe birth practices to traditional birth attendants, health workers and other community leaders.

Between 1988 and 1992, tetanus toxoid immunization of Thai women nearly doubled to 72%, while tetanus shots and boosters were given to nine out of ten schoolchildren. Safe delivery kits were widely distributed, especially where tetanus was most prevalent.

As a result, in the two provinces registering the highest neonatal tetanus rates, the number of cases was halved in three years. □

veys show that one pregnancy in five in the developing world is unwanted when today's communications and outreach capacity is clearly capable of putting the advantages of family planning at the disposal of almost every couple?

In addition, questions were also being raised about one subject which had received very little attention and in which very little progress appeared to have been made. Why, it was asked at the United Nations Safe Motherhood Conference in 1989, were 500,000 young women still dying every year in childbirth in the developing world? Why, for example, were women in sub-Saharan Africa still facing a 1-in-20 risk of dying in childbirth when the risk for a woman in the industrialized world had been reduced to about 1 in 3,600?[19]

New goals

The achievement of the 80% immunization goal galvanized this process. The attainment of this one goal – which for the first time in history brought a basic scientific advance to virtually every community in the world – demonstrated that many other similar and equally important goals could be achieved *if* nations decided to make the attempt and *if* the international community gave its sustained support.

In the fall of 1990, this rising awareness of what could be done culminated in the convening of the first global summit ever held to discuss a major social issue as opposed to political, military, or economic affairs. The World Summit for Children, held at the United Nations in New York, was attended by representatives of almost every nation, including 71 Presidents and Prime Ministers. Its aim was to consider a broad range of advances that had been made possible by advances in knowledge and technology, by reductions in costs, and by the increasing communications capacity in the developing world. The result was a range of new social goals and an agreement – now signed by 159 countries – that each nation would adapt the goals to its own circumstances and draw up a national programme of action for achieving the goals by the year 2000.[20]

Briefly, those new goals include a one-third reduction in under-five mortality rates, the halving of child malnutrition, the achievement of 90% immunization coverage, the control of major childhood diseases, the eradication of polio, the halving of maternal mortality rates, a primary school education for at least 80% of children, the provision of safe water and sanitation for all communities, and the making available of family planning information and services to all who need them.

These targets are another way of expressing the fact that some of the most basic benefits of progress could and should now be made available not just to some but to all. They represent the kind of fundamental improvements in survival, health, and nutrition which the majority of the world already takes for granted. And there is now no good reason to deny these improvements to any family or community no matter where they may live. Although poverty and underdevelopment make the task more difficult, the achievement of these goals does not depend upon sophisticated technologies or expensive professional services; they are, in the main, capable of being reached over the next few years by any developing country that gives the task sufficient priority.

The total extra cost of reaching all of these year 2000 goals is estimated at approximately $25 billion a year. This is a small price to pay for a programme that would effectively protect almost all the world's children from the worst effects of poverty. And it is a price which could be easily afforded if even 20% of present government spending in the developing world, and 20% of overseas aid budgets, were to be allocated to long-term investment in meeting basic human needs for adequate nutrition, primary health care, basic education, safe water supply, and family planning.

At present only about 10% of government spending and of overseas aid budgets is devoted to these purposes.

Fig. 6 Iodine deficiency

Percentage of school-age children with goitre (enlargement of the thyroid gland caused by iodine deficiency).

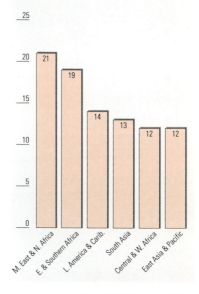

Source: *WHO*, Global prevalence of iodine deficiency disorders, *1993*.

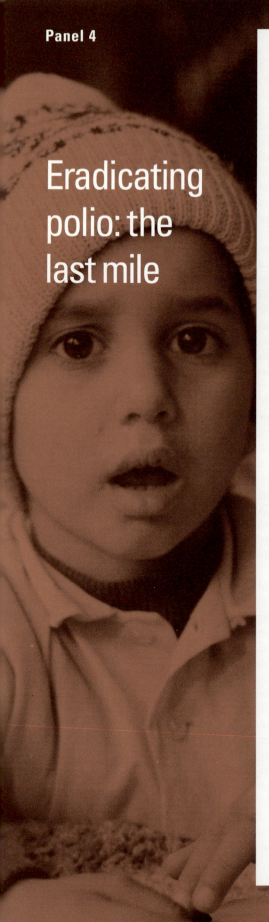

Eradicating polio: the last mile

In 1971, the western hemisphere witnessed its last case of smallpox, foreshadowing global eradication of the disease towards the end of that decade. Twenty years later, in 1991, the Americas offered another good omen to the world as health officials in Peru recorded what they hope will prove the region's last case of endemic polio.

Success in the Americas, along with the rapid rise in polio immunization in the rest of the world, has made great inroads into the territory held by a virus that has crippled uncounted tens of millions of children in this century. In response, the leaders of almost all nations, meeting three years ago at the 1990 World Summit for Children, pledged their best efforts to eradicate polio from the face of the earth by the year 2000.

In the Americas, the battle to eradicate endemic polio transmission began in 1985 – despite the economic and political crises and conflicts confronting so many nations of the region at that time. The effort was spearheaded by the Pan American Health Organization (PAHO), which coordinated government efforts to isolate the polio virus through routine vaccination, national vaccination days, and 'mop-up' operations to contain outbreaks. A network of diagnostic laboratories was also established across the region, along with 20,000 local surveillance centres.

Once the political commitment was made, results came quickly. Brazil, which in 1986 accounted for two thirds of the western hemisphere's 920 polio cases, eliminated the virus within three years. The total cost of the Americas campaign was estimated at $500 million, 80% of it funded by the countries involved.

Polio-free zones are also now emerging in Europe, the Arabian peninsula, the Pacific basin and broad areas of northern, eastern and southern Africa.

Yet no child in any corner of the world is safe from the scourge of polio until the last case has been recorded.

Worldwide immunization coverage – which usually means three doses of vaccine before a child's first birthday – has risen from less than 5% in 1970 to approximately 80% in 1990. Over the past 15 years, the global total of reported cases has dropped from a high of 60,000 in 1982 to around 14,500 for 1992, a clear sign of change even though many polio cases go unreported. The number of countries reporting no endemic cases of polio in 1992 increased to 138, compared with 129 in 1991. The number that have been polio-free for three or more years has risen from 102 in 1991 to 109 in 1992.

As the race to eradicate polio enters the home stretch, there are some signs that the energy is flagging. Global immunization against polio is down slightly from 85% in 1991 to under 80% in 1992. Polio cases were up 40% across South-East Asia in 1992, raising the estimated worldwide number of polio cases in that year from 126,000 to 140,000. Bangladesh, India and Pakistan account for about two thirds of the victims.

Some Governments also failed to submit data on polio to WHO in 1992, and the funding available worldwide has dwindled.

WHO estimates that a total of $1.1 billion will be needed to eradicate polio by the year 2000. As much as two thirds of that cost will have to be borne by the developing world. But it is an investment that would quickly pay off: the savings in vaccination expenses alone will amount to $500 million a year by the end of the century.

The savings in human suffering would be immeasurable. Routine vaccination now spares 400,000 children each year from polio, but the virus still condemns more than 100,000 a year to paralysis of limb and lung. □

National action

Between September 1990 and July 1993, 86 governments have drawn up national programmes of action for reaching the new goals. These programmes are now being put into effect with varying degrees of commitment and funding (panel 7). Another 56 countries are in the final stages of drawing up such plans.

To maintain a sense of urgency, most of the developing world's governments have also agreed to try to reach a limited number of those goals by the middle of the decade. Those 1995 targets include the elimination of neonatal tetanus, a 95% reduction in measles deaths, the promotion of ORT to 80% of the developing world's families, the observance of the WHO/UNICEF code of practice on breastfeeding in the majority of hospitals and maternity units, the elimination of guinea worm disease, the eradication of polio in selected countries, an end to vitamin A deficiency on today's scale, the universal iodization of salt supplies, and the achievement of 80% immunization levels in all countries that have not yet reached that goal.

Reaching these goals would prevent the deaths of over 2 million children a year and protect millions more against major causes of blindness and disability. Yet with the exception of those countries most severely affected by political turbulence or economic decline, including some of the very poorest countries of sub-Saharan Africa, all of these goals are practical and affordable.

When so much could be done for so many and at so little cost, then one central, shameful fact becomes unavoidable: the reason that these problems are not being rapidly overcome is not because the task is too large, or too difficult, or too expensive. It is because the job is not being given sufficient priority. And it is not being given sufficient priority primarily because those most severely affected are almost exclusively the poorest and least politically influential people on earth.

In severity and scale, the cumulative effects of this neglect must be seen as the greatest ethical flaw in our civilization. And like all ethical fault lines, it is likely to result in earthquakes of practical consequences. Part 2 of this report argues that if these problems continue to be ignored, then they are likely to cause ever-worsening problems of social division, political instability, and environmental degradation. The alternative is the use of every possible democratic means to raise the profile and the priority of these issues in order to achieve the great goals that are now so clearly within reach. What is required is a long-term commitment to this cause by political leaders and governments, created or reinforced by pressure from the non-governmental organizations, the media, the professional and business organizations, the religious orders, the academic community, and the public in both industrialized and developing nations.

One measure of that commitment will be the amount of additional resources made available. To reach the agreed goals, it will be necessary to move rapidly to the point at which at least 20% of government expenditures and at least 20% of aid for development are specifically devoted to meeting minimum human needs for adequate nutrition, primary health care, basic education, safe water supply, and family planning.

Making progress

In some key areas, there is already considerable practical progress to report towards the goals for the mid-decade and the year 2000:

☐ The gains made in immunization have, in the main, been sustained and in many cases built upon since 1990. Out of 101 countries for which 1992 figures are available, 37 have increased immunization coverage for completing the third dose of triple vaccine (diphtheria, whooping cough, and tetanus), 30 have maintained the 1990 level, and 34 have fallen back by more than 5 percentage points.[21] Among the developing countries, the year 2000 goal of 90% immunization coverage has already

The job is not being given sufficient priority because those most seriously affected are the poorest and least influential people on earth.

13

been reached in Chile, China, Costa Rica, Cuba, the Democratic People's Republic of Korea, Honduras, Hong Kong, Indonesia, Jordan, Kuwait, Malaysia, Mauritius, Mexico, Oman, the Philippines, Saudi Arabia, Tunisia, and Uruguay.

☐ The mid-decade target of a 90% reduction in measles cases, and a 95% reduction in measles deaths, is likely to be reached in several countries including Brazil, Chile, China, Costa Rica, Rwanda, Tunisia, Viet Nam, and Zimbabwe.[22] Overall, there has already been a 66% reduction in measles cases and an 88% reduction in measles deaths compared to pre-immunization levels.[23]

☐ There is also solid progress to report in the battle to eradicate polio in selected areas by 1995. There have been no new cases of polio in North, Central or South America for the last two years, and polio-free zones are now also being created in Europe, North Africa, Southern Africa and the Middle East. Globally, the number of polio cases has been reduced by approximately 80% compared to pre-immunization levels (fig. 3).[24]

☐ Many nations have now begun to use immunization systems to distribute vitamin A capsules to children over the age of six months – including Bangladesh, Brazil, India, Malawi and the Philippines.[25] In two of the developing world's most populous countries, Bangladesh and India, between 20% and 25% of children have so far been reached. An acceleration of progress – and the use of the immunization system for vitamin A distribution in many more countries – will be necessary if the global target of controlling vitamin A deficiency by 1995 is to be met. Independent reviews conducted in 1992 confirm that, in many areas of the developing world, vitamin A supplements can reduce child deaths by an average of 25%.

☐ Rapid progress is also being made, in many nations, towards the mid-decade goal of eliminating iodine deficiency (panel 8). Over the last five years, national salt iodization programmes have gone into full operation in a total of 24 developing countries –

There have been no new cases of polio in the western hemisphere for the last two years.

including Bangladesh, China, India and Pakistan, which together contain nearly half the developing world's children. By 1995, Bangladesh, China, India and Tanzania will be producing enough iodized salt to protect their entire populations.[26] A further 33 countries are in the process of setting up such programmes.

In some nations, the results are already becoming apparent: Bhutan, Bolivia, and Ecuador, for example, are close to the point of preventing any new cases of iodine deficiency disorders, including cretinism.

☐ The 1990s have also seen continued progress in turning the tide against the bottle-feeding of infants. After more than a decade of work by WHO, UNICEF, and many non-governmental organizations, the free or subsidized distribution of infant formulas to new mothers in hospitals and maternity clinics has been banned in nearly 80 developing countries where the practice was formerly accepted.[27] Under the WHO/UNICEF 'baby-friendly hospital initiative', many hundreds of hospitals and maternity units in over 100 developing and industrialized countries have adopted the 'ten steps to successful breastfeeding' drawn up by WHO and UNICEF in 1989.[28] In hospitals where records have been analysed, the frequency of illness and death among newborns has been substantially reduced and significant financial savings have been made.[29] Given the support of health professionals, the cooperation of infant formula manufacturers, and the continued involvement of the public and the non-governmental organizations, it should be possible to achieve the mid-decade goal of ensuring that the majority of the world's hospitals and maternity units support the exclusive breastfeeding of infants in the first few months of life.

☐ The goal of controlling guinea worm disease by 1995 is also clearly within reach – offering hope to those who suffer months of crippling pain, fever, nausea, vomiting, diarrhoea and general body weakness. Towards the end of the 1980s, the worldwide number of cases of guinea worm disease was estimated at approximately 10 million. The figures for 1992 suggest that the number is now down to fewer than 1 million – 90% of them in just seven African countries. India, where the number of reported cases is down from 40,000 in 1984 to under 1,000 cases in 1992, is on the way to eradicating the disease by 1995. Pakistan reported only 23 cases in 1992 and should soon join the Gambia, Guinea, Guinea-Bissau, Iran, Saudi Arabia, and Yemen on the list of countries that have recently freed themselves of this disease.[30] Two of the worst-affected countries, Ghana and Nigeria, have reduced the number of cases by 50% in the last three years.*

☐ Many developing countries are also making steady and largely unsung progress towards the goal of clean water supply for all communities by the year 2000 (fig. 7). In India, the percentage of rural people with access to safe water has risen from just over 30% in 1980 to over 80% in 1992. If this progress is maintained, then India will reach the year 2000 target of universal access, in rural areas, by 1997. In total, 2.2 million India Mark II handpumps, developed through cooperation between the Government of India, UNICEF, and non-governmental organizations, are now supplying water to over 550 million people at an initial cost of approximately $4 per person.

In Bangladesh, despite all the problems that have been endured since independence, 20 years of determined efforts have succeeded in bringing tube-well drinking water to within 150 metres of 80% of the population (panel 9).

Falling behind

These are considerable achievements. But there are other equally basic benefits of progress which are becoming available much too slowly:

☐ Progress is too slow in reducing deaths from pneumonia – now the biggest single killer of the world's children. Pilot studies in a dozen nations have shown that pneumonia deaths can be reduced by up to 50% if parents are informed of the early danger signs, and if community health workers are

trained in the appropriate use of antibiotics.[31] But although 60 countries are reported to have drawn up plans for action against pneumonia,[32] there is as yet little sign of action *on the necessary scale*. The result is that more than 3 million children are still being allowed to die each year because this relatively simple and inexpensive benefit of modern science has not been made available to the children of the poorest communities. Many complicated, costly, useless, and harmful drugs continue to be marketed and to reach into every village and neighbourhood in the developing world. Yet the cheap and simple antibiotics required to attack the biggest single killer of the world's children are not being made available to those who need them.

☐ Progress in promoting knowledge of ORT has also been too slow. A quarter of a century has now passed since the discovery was made that dehydration could be prevented and treated by a mixture of sugar and salts – a discovery that was described in the 1970s as *"one of the greatest medical breakthroughs of the twentieth century"*.[33] The technique is virtually cost-free. Yet it is still known to only about one third of the developing world's families. And diarrhoeal disease is still killing almost 3 million children a year. If those children were the sons and daughters of better-off or more influential parents, then it is difficult to imagine them dying at such a rate 25 years after the discovery of an effective and low-cost remedy. Some countries, such as Bhutan, Cameroon, Cuba, Iran, Libya, Nigeria, Syria, the United Arab Emirates, Tanzania, Uruguay, Venezuela, and Zambia, have made rapid progress. But in the next two years, an enormous effort must be made in all regions to lift the ORT usage rate to at least 80% (fig. 8).

As with pneumonia, the struggle to protect children against dehydration is largely a struggle to replace bad therapy with good; according to WHO estimates, over $1 billion a year is currently being spent on antidiarrhoeal drugs, most of which are useless or harmful, when all that is needed, in the

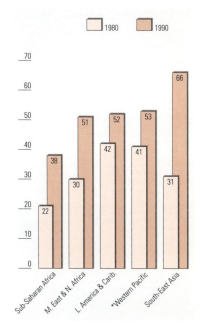

Fig. 7 Safe water

Percentage of people with access to safe water in the rural areas of the developing world.

☐ 1980   ☐ 1990

Region	1980	1990
Sub-Saharan Africa	22	38
M. East & N. Africa	30	51
L. America & Carib.	42	52
*Western Pacific	41	53
South-East Asia	31	66

*Excluding China.

Data for 1980 are only available for the regional groupings as used by the World Health Organization. The figures used in the chart may therefore differ from figures used in the text and statistical tables.

Source: *WHO, unpublished data. Breakdown by WHO regions.*

* If the goal of eradicating guinea worm disease is reached, this particular achievement will owe much to the work of former United States President Jimmy Carter, and to the Carter Center in Atlanta, Georgia, USA, which has rallied international expertise and assistance to this cause for the last six years.

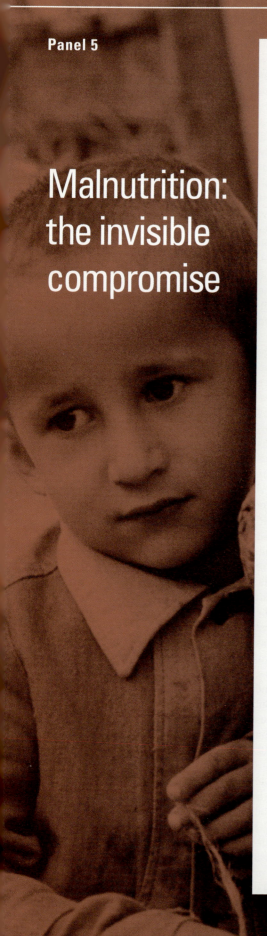

Malnutrition: the invisible compromise

The world's most profound nutritional emergency is not seen on television screens and does not provoke public outrage. Yet common, everyday malnutrition is shocking in both scale and severity; a stealthy accomplice of poverty, it stunts the mental and physical growth of one in three children in the developing world.

Only 1% or 2% of the world's children exhibit visible signs of malnutrition. But an estimated 190 million children under age five are chronically malnourished, locked early into a pattern of ill health and poor development. The problem is most widespread in South Asia, home to half the world's malnourished children.

The ecology of malnutrition is complex. Many households in poor neighbourhoods run short of food between harvests, or amid drought and war. Yet most malnourished children live in homes with adequate food supplies. Only a very small proportion of a family's total food intake is required to feed a young child adequately.

Specific problems such as low birth weight and specific practices such as bottle-feeding contribute heavily to malnutrition. Its principal cause, however, is the constellation of disease, especially diarrhoea, that thrives in poor communities lacking clean water and sanitation. Chronic illness drains nutrients from the body and its cells.

When nourishment runs low, the human body makes compromises to keep going. Mostly, these compromises are invisible – or visible only later to those with growth charts to measure the rate of stunting. Virtually the only outward sign is sluggishness, as the body struggles to conserve energy. Undernourished children stand rather than run and play, sit rather than stand, lie instead of sit.

To compensate for fewer nutrients, the body's metabolic rate drops. Blood pressure sinks. If body fat is low, it 'borrows' from its reserves – depleting muscle instead of fat and slowing or deforming bone growth.

Long before malnutrition becomes visible, it amplifies the worst consequences of illness. The risk of dying from a given disease is doubled for mildly malnourished children, and tripled for those moderately malnourished. In total, it is a factor in one third of the 13 million under-five deaths each year. Good nutrition, on the other hand, is excellent armour against disease.

For a variety of reasons that scientists are only beginning to understand, malnutrition strikes hardest in the last trimester of pregnancy and during the first 12 months after birth. During this vulnerable stage, the tiny stomach requires constant feeding, brain development is nearing completion and the fledgling immune system is weakest.

The most severe effects of stunting are concentrated before a child's first birthday. Even if nutrition improves thereafter, the child is likely to suffer from below-normal growth, affecting physical and mental development and compromising the future of children and their nations.

Poorly nourished mothers tend to give birth to underweight babies – malnourished in the womb and likely to remain so in the crucial early years of life.

At the 1990 World Summit for Children, political leaders agreed on the goal of halving severe and moderate malnutrition rates among under-fives by the year 2000. Large-scale programmes in both Africa and India have recently shown that this can be done.

Even in the midst of an economic crisis, Tanzania's community-based Iringa nutrition programme has more than halved the rate of severe malnutrition in three years. The initial cost of the programme was approximately $16 a child in 1984. That cost has been reduced to about $2.50 per child as the programme goes nationwide. ☐

vast majority of cases, is simple and inexpensive ORT.

☐ The goal of eliminating neonatal tetanus by 1995 will not be reached on present trends (panel 3). In 1990, an estimated 55% of pregnant women in the developing world were immunized against tetanus. By 1993, that figure had fallen to below 40%.[34] If 80% of children can be vaccinated against measles, then there is no reason for the vaccination of women against tetanus to linger at a little over half of that level. Tetanus toxoid vaccine has been available for more than 30 years. Yet the disease is still killing a newborn baby every minute and a new mother every ten minutes.

As with many of the basic benefits of progress reflected in the goals for the year 2000, low levels of coverage with tetanus vaccine can no longer be attributed solely to poverty. Today, success is far more a question of political determination and commitment: India, for example, is one of the poorest countries in the world with a per capita GNP of only $330 a year; yet it has succeeded in immunizing nearly 80% of pregnant women against tetanus. And once the commitment is made, progress can be rapid: Thailand, has cut neonatal tetanus deaths by half in the last three years by training midwives in safe delivery techniques and by doubling its immunization coverage among pregnant women.

☐ There is also little sign of significant progress against maternal mortality. Every year, an estimated 500,000 women die from causes related to pregnancy and childbirth. The goal of halving that toll could be achieved by action on three fronts.

The first is increased investment in family planning services. A disproportionate number of deaths during pregnancy and childbirth are the deaths of women who are too young to give birth safely, or who do not wish to become pregnant, or who seek illegal and unsafe abortions. Family planning could therefore prevent perhaps as many as one quarter of all maternal deaths.

The second step is the provision of basic antenatal care and trained help during delivery. Check-ups during pregnancy can help to detect high blood pressure, anaemia, and malaria (all major causes of maternal death). Two injections can also protect both mother and child against tetanus. During childbirth, all women should be attended by a trained person who can ensure the 'three cleans' (clean hands, clean delivery surface, clean cutting and dressing of the cord) and recognize the signs which mean that more qualified help is needed. At present, only about half of all births in the developing world are attended by a trained person.

The third step is the provision of emergency obstetric care for women who encounter problems after childbirth has begun. This does not usually require advanced technologies or expensive facilities. It can normally be provided at relatively low cost by existing district hospitals and maternity units. Every family should therefore be aware of the risks of childbirth. And every father-to-be should try to make preparations – in advance – for transport to a hospital or maternity unit should the need arise.

Achieving the goal of a 50% reduction in maternal mortality by the end of the century is therefore not impossible at present levels of economic development. It would imply bringing the average maternal mortality rate down to approximately 150 deaths per 100,000 births – a level already achieved by several of the poorest countries in the world, including China, the Democratic People's Republic of Korea, Mongolia, the Philippines, Sri Lanka, Viet Nam, and Zambia.[35]

☐ Progress is also too slow in education. The goal of providing a primary education for at least 80% of children is one of the most important of all the goals for the development of individuals and of nations – but it is also one of the most difficult to achieve. After making rapid gains in the 1960s and 1970s, primary school enrolment and retention levels have stagnated or fallen in a number of developing countries, particularly in sub-Saharan Africa, during the last decade.

In almost all regions, the problem is

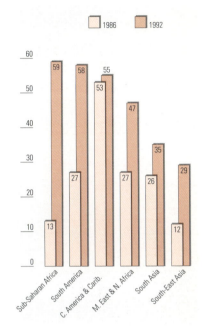

Fig. 8 Oral rehydration

Percentage of diarrhoea episodes treated with oral rehydration therapy (ORT).

☐ 1986   ☐ 1992

ORT includes both the use of oral rehydration salts and/or recommended fluids for rehydration. The range of recommended fluids varies from country to country.

Source: *WHO, unpublished.*

one of retention as well as enrolment: over 90% of the developing world's children already enrol in grade 1 of primary school, but less than two thirds of those enrolled stay at school for as long as four years.

☐ Progress in making family planning available to all couples is also being slowed in some countries by lack of funds and lack of priority. Recent achievements have been extraordinary, but they have also been uneven: access to family planning services has reached 95% in East Asia (including China), over 60% in South-East Asia and Latin America, about 55% in South Asia, and less than 10% in Africa.[36]

In sub-Saharan Africa, in particular, the problem goes much deeper than lack of priority and lack of funds. High child death rates and low levels of education for women mean that *demand* for family planning remains lower than elsewhere. Meanwhile health budgets have suffered disproportionately as a result of debt, adjustment policies, and falling commodity prices – with the result that the *supply* of family planning information and services has also suffered.

Lack of data

Finally, there is as yet no very significant progress in putting in place the data-collection systems needed to monitor progress in all of these basic areas of human progress. Many countries produce quarterly statistics on the health and growth of their economies; very few produce even annual statistics on the health and growth of their children. Yet such statistics are essential for informing policy, for strengthening accountability, and for generating informed public and political debate.

In all countries, academic institutions, non-governmental organizations, professional bodies, the business community, and the media have a responsibility to ensure that such statistics are widely known and used. Economic statistics now feature regularly in all serious media and have become a normal part of political life in almost all nations; if the task of bringing basic advantages of progress to all is to be given more priority, then similar use must now be made of statistics which show the proportion of a nation's children that remains malnourished, or uneducated, or unimmunized, or dies from preventable illnesses, or lacks access to safe water supplies.

As one contribution to this monitoring process, UNICEF has this year launched a new publication – *The Progress of Nations* – which uses the latest available statistics to record and compare national achievements in child survival, health, nutrition, education, family planning, and progress for women.[37]

Not by GNP alone

Of the most basic, low-cost, life-improving advances that ought to be available to all families, only immunization has so far reached a majority of the poorest billion people on earth.

In part, the problem is a residual belief that these problems are too big and too expensive to be overcome at the present time, a widespread feeling that 'the poor will always be with us'. But with each year that passes, it becomes more and more clear that controlling the worst aspects of poverty is not a question of possibilities but of priorities.

Two arguments substantiate this view. First, the significant progress of recent years has, by and large, been achieved by a comparatively low level of commitment by governments. It has already been mentioned that the developing world's governments spend only about 10% of their budgets on meeting basic human needs for nutrition, water supply, primary health care, primary education, and family planning.[38] Similarly, the proportion of bilateral aid that is specifically devoted to long-term investment in meeting these minimum human needs is also about 10%.[39] Less than 2.5% of aid, for example, goes to primary education, and only about 1.5% goes to family planning.[40]

Such figures reflect the low level of priority that policy makers have given to the task of bringing the most basic

High child death rates and low levels of education for women mean that demand for family planning remains low.

benefits of progress to the poorest quarter of the world's people, and it is reasonable to assume that if the task had been given a significantly higher priority over the last two decades, nationally and internationally, then it would by now have been largely accomplished.

Secondly, there is the evidence of those countries which, although still struggling at relatively low levels of economic development, have nonetheless made very significant strides towards bringing basic benefits of progress to all their citizens. Many poor countries are today closer to meeting the most basic needs of their peoples than other countries that are considerably wealthier. Eight of the poorest countries in the world, with per capita incomes below $1,000 a year and a wide range of different political systems, have already reached the goal of reducing under-five mortality rates to 70 per 1,000 births or less: China, the Democratic People's Republic of Korea, the Dominican Republic, Egypt, Honduras, the Philippines, Sri Lanka, and Viet Nam.

Similarly, several of the poorest nations in the world, including four in sub-Saharan Africa, have already reduced malnutrition rates below 15% – less than half the average rate for the developing world as a whole.[41]

Many countries with per capita GNPs of less than $1,000 a year have also surpassed the 80% immunization mark, while other nations with twice that level of GNP still linger at considerably lower levels.

In the field of education, China, Indonesia, Sri Lanka, and Zimbabwe have all reached the goal of providing at least four years of primary school for at least 80% of their children, despite being among the poorest of the world's countries.

Promises and pressure

These examples, along with the recent achievements already discussed, show how remarkable is the present potential. The technologies and strategies for bringing basic benefits of progress to all peoples are now available and affordable. The communications and outreach capacity is, by and large, in place. Clear goals have been established and agreed upon by the great majority of the world's political leaders. And all of this is happening against a backdrop of the end of the cold war, the accession of a new generation of leaders in the United States, the beginning of a fall in military spending in almost all regions, and the faltering but unmistakable worldwide move towards greater participation and democracy of the kind that must ultimately augur well for improvements in the lives of large numbers of the poorest people in the developing world.[42]

Taken together, all of these factors may mean that the world is about to fulfil the promise held out by the historian Arnold Toynbee who wrote, in the years before the cold war descended upon the world, that "*Our age is the first generation since the dawn of history in which mankind dared to believe it practical to make the benefits of civilization available to the whole human race.*"

Public pressure

The immediate threat to this great hope is that the commitments that have been made will not command a sufficient and sustained priority. Issues which are long term, and of primary interest to the poor, have always perched precariously on national and international agendas. And it is when the summit meetings and conferences are over, and the declarations and the promises have been made, that the wider battle must begin to maintain those commitments in the face of more immediate issues and more powerful interest groups.

Sustained support and pressure from a broad public, and especially from the non-governmental organizations, from the media, from political and religious leaders, from professional bodies and business leaders, and from the academic community, is therefore essential if the commitments that have been made are to be given content and impetus. Standing alone,

Many poor countries are today closer to meeting the most basic needs of their peoples than other countries that are considerably wealthier.

19

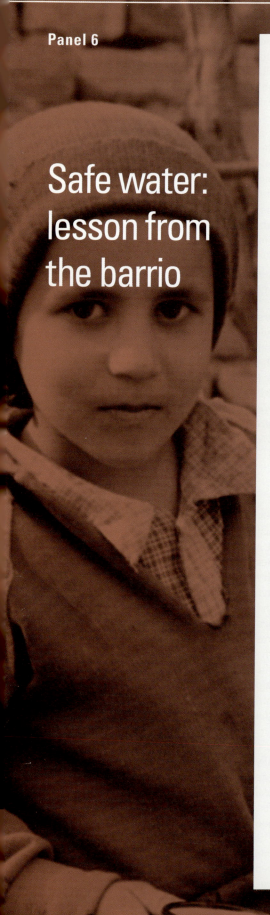

Safe water: lesson from the barrio

The cities of the developing world are growing three times as fast as rural areas. Within 15 years, half the developing world's population will be urban. Cities will have to double the capacity of basic services like water and sanitation simply to maintain the status quo.

Tegucigalpa, the capital of Honduras, offers an example of both the problem and a promising solution. In 20 years, its population has trebled to 750,000 as migrants from the countryside have come in search of jobs. Two thirds of them live in the shanty towns known as *barrios marginales*.

Most barrio dwellers buy water for washing and drinking from private vendors. The water is often unsafe, and they pay ten times as much per gallon as residents who are connected to the public water system. Lack of adequate water and safe sanitation means frequent illness and poor growth: one in ten children dies before reaching the age of five – a third of the deaths being from diarrhoeal disease.

In 1987, the Honduran national water and sanitation agency, with UNICEF support, launched an innovative programme using independent wells, communal tanks, and trucks to provide water in poor neighbourhoods. Within five years, more than 50,000 people in 26 barrios were getting water from safe, reliable and permanent sources, cutting annual household water expenditure from 40% of income to only 4%.

The cornerstone of the Honduras strategy is the community water board elected by each barrio. Boards recruit volunteer labour, manage and maintain the water system, send bills to users and, ultimately, repay the investment made by UNICEF and the Government. In a parallel UNICEF project, many families showed willingness to pay for decent sanitation by taking out – and repaying – loans to build sanitary units.

By means of such strategies – including community participation, cost sharing, and cost recovery – universal access to clean water and sanitation can be achieved by the end of the century. The cost of drilling wells and installing pumps is no longer prohibitive. A decade ago it cost $9,500 to sink a handpump-equipped borehole in the Sudan. Today, that cost is down to $2,800.

But it is equally obvious that the goal of universal access will not be achieved by current strategies.

Of the estimated $10 billion a year spent by governments and aid-giving countries on water supply, only about $2 billion is helping to finance schemes like the one in Honduras which provide a low-cost service based on handpump-equipped boreholes and street or yard water-standpipes serving primarily the poor. The other $8 billion is allocated to relatively high-cost systems – water treatment plants, pumping stations, individual household water supply, and highly mechanized sewage systems – serving mostly the better-off communities. Most governments are also subsidizing the operation and maintenance costs by as much as 70%.

Approximately 1.2 billion people in the developing world are today denied access to a bare minimum of safe drinking water. On present patterns of progress, an estimated 770 million people will still be without safe water by the end of the century, and the number of people without adequate sanitation will have increased to approximately 1.9 billion.

The message of the last decade could not be clearer. The year 2000 goal of making safe water and sanitation available to all can be achieved – but only by restructuring government expenditures and international aid in favour of low-cost community-based strategies for the poorest. □

the formal commitments of political leaders to internationally agreed goals, and the drawing up of national programmes of action, are not enough.

In the industrialized nations, in particular, there is a desperate need for restructuring aid programmes so that at least 20% of aid is allocated to meeting the minimum human needs of the poorest people. Investment in basic health, nutrition, education, and employment opportunities is the kind of aid which the majority of people in the industrialized world wish to give,[43] and the kind of aid which the majority of people in the developing world wish to receive. But to a large extent, the size and shape of today's aid programmes remain frozen in the pattern of the cold war era. About 25% of United States foreign assistance is military aid and for fiscal year 1994 more than 25% of non-military aid is earmarked for Egypt, Israel, and the nations of the former Soviet Union – leaving only about $6.5 billion for the rest of the developing world. In addition to such foreign policy imperatives, aid is also distorted by the weight of history and of commercial considerations. Only about 25% of all aid, for example, goes to the ten countries in the world that are home to 75% of the world's poor.[44]

At a time when many had hoped that the end of the cold war would unfreeze substantial financial resources for addressing some of the most basic problems of world poverty, the international development effort is in fact facing a severe financial crisis. The enormous demand for aid and investment in Eastern Europe and the countries of the former Soviet Union, combined with unprecedented deficits in several major industrialized countries and the increased cost of peacekeeping activities in such 'failed states' as Somalia and former Yugoslavia, means that the poorest countries of the world are being deprived of aid, loans, and investments at the same time as they are also being squeezed by debt obligations and by falling prices for the raw commodities on which their economies still largely depend.

To ease this financial famine, and to support the developing world in reaching the basic human goals that have been agreed, will demand considerable vision on the part of leaders in industrialized nations. But it will also require the courage and tenacity to hold fast to that vision in the face of all the immediate problems and pressures crowding the agendas of political leaders in the 1990s.

The 21st century

Over and above the problems of priority and resources, the process of bringing the most basic benefits of progress to all communities is confronted by a long-term threat of even greater magnitude. There is a clear and growing danger that both present potential and past achievements may be overwhelmed, in the years ahead, by the growing crises of absolute poverty, rapid population growth, and increasing environmental pressures. As this 'PPE problem' intensifies, the task of realizing today's potential for bringing the most basic benefits of progress to all peoples may be afforded even less priority than in the recent past. This would represent not only an inhuman response, but also a profoundly mistaken one. For the achievement of basic human goals is not only a humanitarian imperative, it is also one of the most powerful and accessible means of strengthening the movement towards democracy, and of pre-empting the great problems that lie ahead.

PPE problems are therefore the unavoidable context of the progress and the potential discussed in part 1 of this report. They are examined in some detail in part 2, in order to show how they might affect, and be affected by, the attempt to bring some of the most basic benefits of progress to all the world's communities in the years to come.

At least 20% of international aid should be allocated to meeting the minimum human needs of the poorest people.

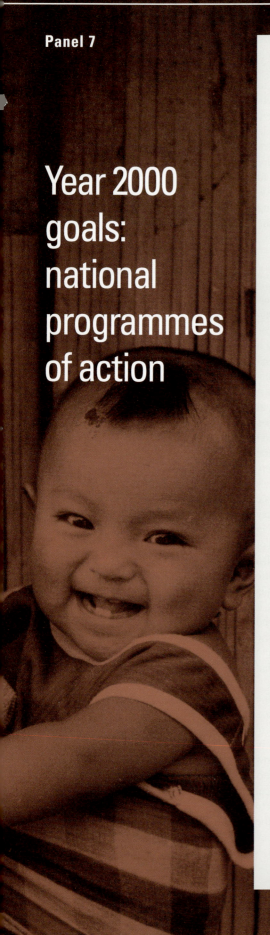

Year 2000 goals: national programmes of action

At the 1990 World Summit for Children, 149 countries formally committed themselves to establishing national programmes of action (NPAs) for achieving the year 2000 goals adopted at the Summit. By July 1993, less than three years after the Summit, 90% of the world's children were living in countries with NPAs finalized or in draft: 86 Governments had completed their programmes and were beginning to implement them.

NPAs offer a new, strategic approach to the somewhat discredited but still necessary task of planning for human development. With their focus on children, they can rise above political divisions and survive changes of regime. Integrated into national development plans, as they are in some of the largest countries such as China, Egypt, India and Indonesia, along with many smaller ones, NPAs provide a focus and a direction for investment in a country's future. They can serve as instruments for increased collaboration between bilateral and multilateral agencies, as a key component to the development of broader programmes for poverty eradication, and as part of a macro-strategy for sustainable development following the guidelines of Agenda 21, the blueprint for the world's environment agreed at the 'Earth Summit' in Rio de Janeiro in 1992.

NPAs are an important instrument for bridging the gap between ratification of the Convention on the Rights of the Child and its implementation. They represent practical, affordable programmes for ensuring a minimum set of children's rights within a reasonable period of time.

NPAs are most dynamic where they have the personal backing of heads of state or government – as in Mexico, whose President has personally taken part in five public evaluations of NPA implementation – and where NPA preparation and implementation have been highly public and broadly participatory – as in the Dominican Republic, where 125 non-governmental organizations form part of the commission responsible for NPA implementation. In Uganda, the National Council for Children includes government, local and international non-governmental groups, religious institutions, donor governments, and concerned individuals.

Brazil's 'Pact for Children' brings together both the legislative and executive branches of government, the National Council of Brazilian Churches, the governors of all 27 states, and key non-governmental organizations.

Many countries are decentralizing the NPA process. State or provincial plans of action are being prepared in such diverse countries as Brazil, Ecuador and Viet Nam. Municipal plans have been drawn up by large cities such as Dakar and Mexico City, as well as by smaller ones such as Khulna in Bangladesh and Rosario in Argentina.

By estimating the resources required to achieve the goals, NPAs help to identify where and to what extent national budgets, and external aid, must be restructured to ensure the fulfilment of priority human development needs. The test lies in finding the resources. Most countries are funding their programmes chiefly by redirecting a larger share of the national budget to social services. In Namibia and Zimbabwe, for example, cut-backs in arms spending are being reallocated to children. Mexico's expenditure per child in 1993 was nearly double the 1989 rate.

Some of the better-off nations of the developing world, like the Republic of Korea, are funding their national programmes on their own. But for many poorer nations, the hopes embodied in their NPAs will only be realized if they receive the help that has been promised by donor nations and the international community. □

The PPE spiral

The collapse of the former Soviet Union and the ending of the bipolar world order have clearly brought an era of history to an end. But the view that the cold war has gone out with a whimper rather than a bang, and that one side has won with hardly a shot being fired, is the first and most dangerous placebo of the new age. The cold war has been more destructive than any war in human history; it has been a war in which there have been no winners, and a war of which the severest consequences may yet be to come.

Apart from the nurturing of military regimes in many parts of the world, with all that this has meant for the abuse of human rights and the neglect of human needs, the chief consequence of the cold war has been the colossal diversion of financial, human, and natural resources to essentially unproductive purposes. Meanwhile, urgent human and environmental problems have been neglected, and have consequently grown in scale and seriousness throughout the cold war era.

The magnitude of this distraction can be roughly gauged by its financial cost: throughout the late 1980s, the world's military spending was running close to one trillion dollars a year,[45] or the equivalent of the combined annual incomes of the poorest half of the world's people.

Yet even this statistic cannot fully encompass the damage done to human history by this 50-year diversion of human energies and ambitions, of scientific research and technological ingenuity, of industrial productivity and organizational capacity. Nor can any figure distil the cost of progress forgone, or display the panoply of what might have been achieved if these resources had been devoted to social and economic progress, to peaceful scientific advance, and to the understanding and protection of the environment. But it may reasonably be assumed that if one half or even one quarter of these colossal resources had been intelligently devoted to such purposes, then we could now be living in a world in which mass hunger, malnutrition, preventable disease, illiteracy, rapid population growth, and a deteriorating global environment would be problems of the past.

As it is, all of these problems have been allowed to assume their present, much less manageable scale. Those problems now include:

☐ The absolute poverty of approximately one fifth of the world's population. A majority of this poorest billion people on earth are people whose environments are being rapidly degraded, and whose lives are becoming increasingly hard and desperate, even as global communications ensure that they are ever more aware of levels of prosperity in the rest of the world;

☐ A rate of population growth which, if present trends continue, will quadruple the numbers of the poor within a single lifetime (fig. 9). In the next 40 years, the population of sub-Saharan Africa is projected to almost treble from approximately 600 million to more than 1.6 billion.[46] Over the same period, the population of Asia will rise from just over 3 billion to just over 5 billion;

☐ A pattern of consumption and pollution in the industrialized nations which cannot long be supported without serious damage to the biosphere, but which cannot long be denied to those far more populous areas of the world that are likely to make rapid economic progress in the years ahead. The industrialized nations, with approximately 20% of the world's people, are currently responsible for three quarters of the world's energy use, two

Fig. 9 Population projections

Present population of the major regions of the world and projected population (in billions) in the year 2100.

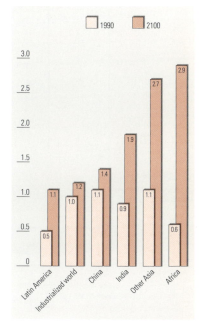

Source: *United Nations*, Long-range world population projections: two centuries of population growth 1950-2150, *1992*.

Fig. 10 Population and pollution

Percentage share of total population and total chlorofluorocarbon (CFC) emissions of the industrialized and developing worlds.

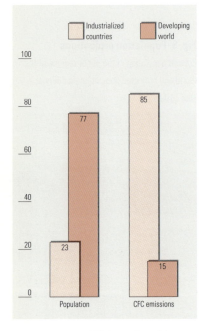

CFCs damage the earth's ozone layer and contribute to global warming.

Source: *World Resources Institute*, World resources 1992-93, *1992.*

thirds of all greenhouse gases, and 90% of the chlorofluorocarbons that threaten the earth's protective ozone layer (fig. 10).[47]

It may well be that these problems have already accumulated to the point at which some degree of disaster is inevitable, and it is in this sense that the true costs of the cold war are still to be revealed. But as human society shuffles free from this historic distraction, the hope must be that the cold war has ended in time for the world to refocus itself, switching its concern and capacities to the task of averting a catastrophe brought on by the neglect and accumulation of these problems during the long years of military and ideological preoccupation.

PPE problems

As individual nations and the international community turn to face these gathering crises, it is the problems facing the poorest fifth of the world's people that are likely to be accorded the lowest priority. Yet that is where the search for solutions must begin.

Within an international economic framework that disables rather than enables the poorest countries and peoples, the principal threat to the world's poorest billion people comes from the interaction of poverty, population growth, and environmental deterioration. As these problems become more and more interrelated, it is becoming essential to see them as one problem. To that end, this discussion of poverty-population-environment uses the single term 'PPE problems', and attempts to maintain a view of the issue as a whole even at the risk of simplifying its component parts. The diagram on page 25 takes this process one stage further by schematizing the main synergisms that make up the PPE spiral – the mutually reinforcing relationships between poverty, population growth, and environmental stress.

The worst aspects of poverty provide the impetus for the PPE spiral. And the first of the mutually reinforcing relationships which it sets up is that between poverty and rising rates of population growth.

Prolonged and rapid population growth is the child of an unsatisfactory encounter between poverty and progress. As the first wave of relatively easy improvements in public health occurs, crude death rates fall. But birth rates remain high for a variable period, during which the gap between birth and death rates is wide and population growth is rapid. Even when birth rates eventually begin to fall, the period of rapid growth has so altered the age structure of populations that the bulk of a nation's people are young and about to enter their child-bearing years. The result is an inbuilt population momentum which means that the absolute number of people continues to rise even after birth rates fall steeply.

The key variable is the length of time that birth rates remain high after crude death rates have fallen. And the engine that maintains high birth rates during this period is the persistence of some of the worst forms of poverty and deprivation:

☐ Lack of progress in health care, which means that child death rates remain high and parents tend to insure against anticipated deaths by having more children;[48]

☐ Lack of status, education, and opportunities for women, a characteristic of most underdeveloped societies, which is strongly associated with early marriage and frequent and prolonged child-bearing;[49]

☐ Lack of minimal security, which makes large families attractive as a potential source of support in illness or old age or in times of danger and emergency;[50]

☐ Lack of investment in basic services and labour-saving technologies, from water-pipes and handpumps to fuel-efficient stoves and grinding mills, which makes large numbers of children desirable, even essential, as a source of help in fields and homes;[51]

☐ Lack of family planning information and services, which often causes birth rates to remain high even when circumstances change and large numbers of people begin to consider the advantages of smaller families;

THE PPE SPIRAL

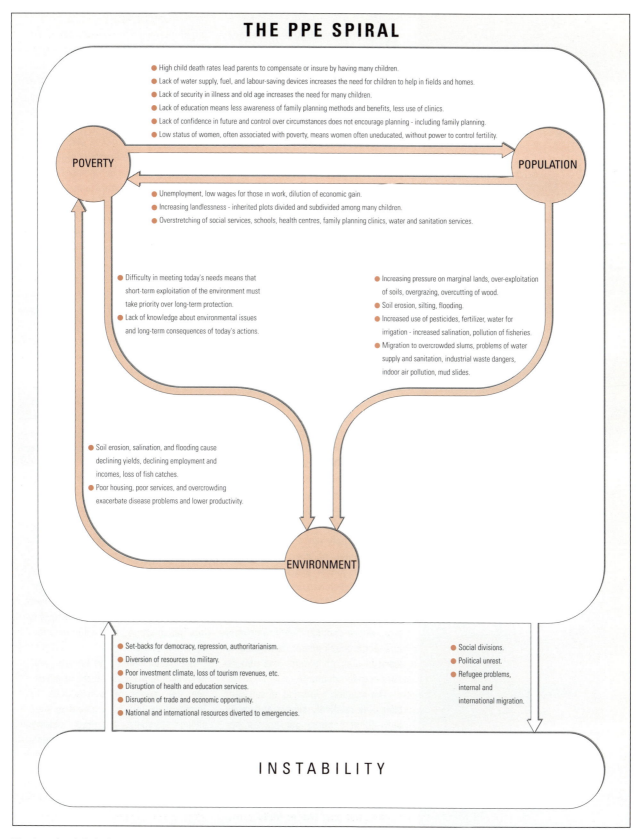

POVERTY

POPULATION

- High child death rates lead parents to compensate or insure by having many children.
- Lack of water supply, fuel, and labour-saving devices increases the need for children to help in fields and homes.
- Lack of security in illness and old age increases the need for many children.
- Lack of education means less awareness of family planning methods and benefits, less use of clinics.
- Lack of confidence in future and control over circumstances does not encourage planning - including family planning.
- Low status of women, often associated with poverty, means women often uneducated, without power to control fertility.

- Unemployment, low wages for those in work, dilution of economic gain.
- Increasing landlessness - inherited plots divided and subdivided among many children.
- Overstretching of social services, schools, health centres, family planning clinics, water and sanitation services.

- Difficulty in meeting today's needs means that short-term exploitation of the environment must take priority over long-term protection.
- Lack of knowledge about environmental issues and long-term consequences of today's actions.

- Increasing pressure on marginal lands, over-exploitation of soils, overgrazing, overcutting of wood.
- Soil erosion, silting, flooding.
- Increased use of pesticides, fertilizer, water for irrigation - increased salination, pollution of fisheries.
- Migration to overcrowded slums, problems of water supply and sanitation, industrial waste dangers, indoor air pollution, mud slides.

- Soil erosion, salination, and flooding cause declining yields, declining employment and incomes, loss of fish catches.
- Poor housing, poor services, and overcrowding exacerbate disease problems and lower productivity.

ENVIRONMENT

- Set-backs for democracy, repression, authoritarianism.
- Diversion of resources to military.
- Poor investment climate, loss of tourism revenues, etc.
- Disruption of health and education services.
- Disruption of trade and economic opportunity.
- National and international resources diverted to emergencies.

- Social divisions.
- Political unrest.
- Refugee problems, internal and international migration.

INSTABILITY

The above chart is limited to processes within the developing world. But the PPE spiral is compounded by the industrialized world's policies in the fields of aid, trade, finance, and debt.

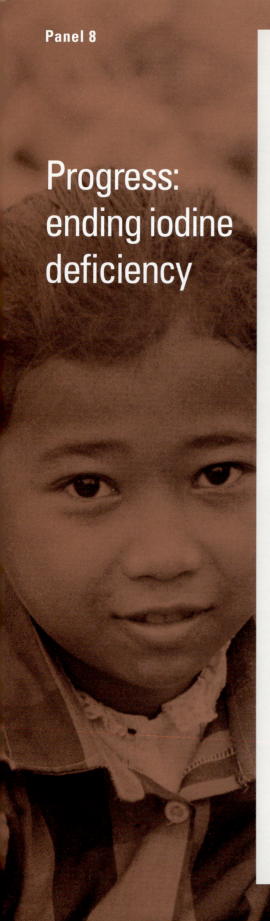

Progress: ending iodine deficiency

Attitudes towards the little-known and much-ignored problem of iodine deficiency are going through a revolution in the 1990s.

Three years ago, at the 1990 World Summit for Children, the world's political leaders promised a new effort to end iodine deficiency disorders by the end of the century. At that time, the true scale and severity of the problem was just beginning to become known outside medical and scientific circles. But since then, the map of the problem has been re-drawn by a series of new surveys and by advances in understanding of the damage that can be done by even mild levels of iodine deficiency.

It is now estimated that nearly 1.6 billion people in over 110 nations are at risk and that some 300 million suffer from lowered mental ability. Some 566 million – about 10% of world population and more than double the previous estimate – suffer from goitre, the tell-tale swelling of the thyroid gland at the throat.

Because their mothers lack iodine, at least 30,000 babies are stillborn every year, and over 120,000 are born cretins – mentally retarded, physically stunted, deaf-mute or paralysed. Many more have IQs at least 10 points below their potential. Even when born normal, young children whose diets are low in iodine are held back by reduced intelligence, and live out their lives trapped in mental dullness and apathy. In this way the lack of iodine locks entire communities into poverty and underdevelopment, less able to learn in their childhood, less able to earn in their adulthood.

The solution – iodizing all salt supplies – is relatively simple and costs only about 5 cents per person per year. Within a year of iodized salt becoming the norm, no more cretins are born and goitres begin to shrink. Children develop energy and perform better at school.

Over the past two or three years, many countries have launched iodizing programmes or reinvigorated their existing efforts, and a worldwide goal of iodizing all salt supplies by the end of 1995 has now been accepted by the leaders of almost all developing nations. Bangladesh, China, India and Tanzania – with nearly half of the world's people at risk – are already well on the way to reaching that goal.

Iodizing salt is comparatively straightforward when it can be done in a single location. In Syria, for instance, the Ministry of Industry is the sole salt producer and has just started iodizing the nation's salt. In Bhutan, where salt is imported over a border crossing from India, an iodizing plant installed at the border a decade ago has brought child goitre rates down from 60% to 25%.

When salt is produced by small-scale entrepreneurs – over 10,000 of them in India alone – the process is more complex. Salt producers must be motivated to iodize their product and package it to retain iodine; meanwhile the public must be educated on the benefits of paying slightly more for treated salt.

Bolivia tackled this problem by setting up a private company to popularize iodized salt. As the demand grew, 35 salt companies took up iodizing, with government help to keep the price down. Bolivian police spot-check the salt's iodine content as it leaves the salt-producing areas. Now, over 80% of the population has access to iodized salt, and the goitre rate has dropped to a third of its original level of 60%.

In India, radio, television and newspapers are being used to advertise the merits of iodized salt. In Bangladesh, the Government is supplying specially designed iodizing machines and packaging equipment, free of charge, to all 265 of the country's salt-crushing factories. Installation will be completed by early-1994. □

☐ Lack of confidence and hope in the future, which is the great enemy of life planning in general and family planning in particular.[52]

In addition to these forces, other powerful if unquantifiable factors have always tended to link poverty with large families: behaviour patterns which were once necessary for protection or survival tend to become entrenched in cultures and traditions that are often slow to change with changing circumstance. And in very poor societies, children may be one of the few sources of joy and pride, of change and hope, in lives that are often monotonous, hard, and resigned.

In sum, poverty is the coiled spring that powers population growth.

Perpetuating poverty

But if poverty provides the impetus to rapid population growth, then population growth, in its turn, provides a new impetus to poverty. This is the first of the major synergisms within the downward spiral of PPE problems.

In the past, high birth rates have often gone hand in hand with high rates of economic growth, and large families have been encouraged by leaders and governments as a means of strengthening nations militarily and economically, providing the state with larger numbers of workers, consumers, taxpayers and soldiers. But in most parts of the developing world today, the circumstances are such that high rates of population growth are serving to perpetuate poverty in a number of obvious ways:

☐ By causing the labour force to grow more quickly than employment opportunities, thereby creating large numbers of unemployed and underemployed people and depressing the wages of those who do find work;

☐ By placing increasing stress on the resources by which the poor make their living and meet their needs in rural areas – soils and soil fertility, fuel supplies and animal fodder, grazing land and water sources;

☐ By causing inherited smallholdings to be divided and subdivided among large numbers of children. Along with gross inequalities in land ownership, this means that many millions of rural people find themselves landless or near-landless, and are thereby unable to meet their needs for food and fuel, work and income;

☐ By reducing the amount of time, care, and resources available for each child;[53]

☐ By reducing the time available to the mother for earning income, or for other economically productive work;

☐ By raising the cost to governments of providing adequate health and education services for the rising generation, and by overstretching schools, clinics, and water and sanitation systems. All of this helps to maintain high levels of malnutrition, disease, and illiteracy, which in turn help to keep communities in poverty;

☐ By causing overcrowding and a lower quality of life in slums and shanty towns, with all the attendant evils of disease, hopelessness, loss of self-respect, breakdown of family ties, weakening of family support, alcohol and drug abuse, increasing violence, and the abandonment of women and children.

In these ways, population growth tends to reinforce poverty, and poverty tends to reinforce population growth, forming a circuit through which the current of poverty's perpetuation flows.

Environmental stress

Increasing environmental pressures are now assuming the proportions of a major crisis in the lives of hundreds of millions of people in the developing world. Several recent studies have explored this relationship between poverty and environmental pressure,[54] and it is only necessary here to stress the mutually reinforcing nature of that relationship and its role in the PPE spiral.

Against a background of poverty, rapidly growing numbers of people are finding themselves without enough land to meet their needs and without any substantial hope of alternative employment. In almost all regions of

Lack of confidence and hope in the future is the great enemy of life planning in general - and family planning in particular.

27

The developing countries that have succeeded have been those that have tackled the task of land reform and invested in the health, nutrition, and education of their people.

the developing world, this fundamental problem of landlessness and unemployment is in large part caused and perpetuated by lack of investment in small farms and by the concentration of productive lands in the hands of a small number of wealthy families or large corporations.

During the first stages of rapid population increase in today's industrialized nations, rising numbers of poor people also suffered from distress in the countryside and destitution in urban slums. But among many other advantages, they had available to them the freedom to industrialize, to export, and to migrate, and were eventually able to absorb or disperse increasing numbers of people who could no longer be sustained by agriculture alone. It is of the greatest significance that this combination of advantages has not, in general, been available to the majority of developing countries during their period of similarly rapid population growth.

In those developing countries that have gone through an agricultural revolution, many millions of people have seen steady and substantial gains in their incomes and standard of living over the past three decades. In the main, those beneficiaries have been people who owned enough of the right land in the right place and who had access to the necessary inputs and credit facilities. But in the absence of land reform, agricultural revolutions tend to result in falling employment per hectare as land ownership becomes more unequal, farms become larger, and large-scale mechanization becomes possible.

At the same time, population growth means that the remaining smallholdings are divided up among larger numbers of children, eventually becoming too small and too fragmented to sustain a family's needs.

The result of both of these forces is that many tens of millions of smallholders, tenant farmers, and agricultural labourers have found themselves without sufficient land or sufficient work. From India to Brazil, uncounted numbers of rural families have become effectively landless or have been turned away from the fields that they once helped to till and harvest.

With some exceptions, the growth of agricultural and industrial employment has usually not been rapid enough to absorb this surplus. In part, this is the result of internal mistakes: ill-judged investments; crippling taxation and exchange-rate policies; large-scale corruption; inefficient state control of large agricultural enterprises; lack of land reform; and the mistaken emphasis on capital-intensive rather than labour-intensive investment policies.

Those developing countries and regions that have succeeded in absorbing growing numbers of people into productive employment have been, by and large, those that have tackled the difficult task of land reform and invested in the health, nutrition, and education of their people. If, like Taiwan and the Republic of Korea, they have also ensured reasonable incentives to farmers, and made available rural credit, farm inputs, and infrastructure, then both employment and productivity per hectare have increased on many thousands of small and medium-size farms. Rising prosperity in rural areas has helped, in turn, to provide markets for, and jobs in, a growing industrial sector.

But in the many developing countries that have failed to institute such reforms and make such investments, the freedom to industrialize has also been circumscribed by forces over which they have little control. Potential markets are dominated by the already industrialized nations, and attempts to export manufactured goods have often been impeded by trade and tariff barriers that restrict the growth of employment and cost the developing world approximately twice as much every year in lost earnings as it receives in aid.[55]

Nor has freedom of external migration been a significant option. Domestic or foreign legislation has permitted only a very small proportion of the developing world's people to travel overseas to seek new opportunities; by and large, those who have been allowed to migrate have been the better-off and the better educated rather than the landless and asset-less poor. During Europe's period of rapid population growth, there were many tens of millions of people who found themselves in a similar position to the landless and jobless poor of the developing world today, but who were able to migrate to new opportunities in Australia, Canada, New Zealand, South Africa and the United States.[56] Between the end of the Napoleonic wars and the beginning of the First World War, for example, 20 million people emigrated from the United Kingdom alone.[57]

The lack of these freedoms, combined with a lack of land reform and a lack of investment in labour-intensive productivity on small farms, has meant that the landless and the jobless of the developing world have tended to migrate internally to one of two destinations: either they have moved onto relatively sparsely populated and previously less valued lands – tropical forests, uncultivated hillsides, less fertile lands, and the fragile margins of deserts – or they have migrated to the informal sector of the towns and cities, finding homes in the slums and shanties erected on lands that are similarly unwanted and unvalued.

The effect of this migration, over time, is that poverty has become more and more concentrated in marginal agricultural lands and in urban slums, two different destinations of which the common characteristic is that they are both environmentally vulnerable.

The inevitable consequence, for many millions of people, has been that poverty and hardship have tended to increase as the precarious resource base of the poor has been steadily degraded. Land cleared by burning forests loses stability and fertility within a very few years; steep hillsides quickly become eroded without investments in soil conservation; marginal agricultural lands gradually become infertile when those who farm them can afford neither fertilizer nor fallow periods; desert margins soon become indistinguishable from deserts when

they are subjected to overcutting of wood and overgrazing by animals. Meanwhile, the millions who have found themselves in urban slums are exposed to the environmental problems of overcrowded and usually insanitary conditions, and to all the environmental dangers of living on land that nobody else wants – land far away from services or employment opportunities, land close to railway lines and airports, land near polluting industries or foul-smelling slaughterhouses, land on steep hillsides in danger from earthquakes and mud slides, land next to fly-infested garbage dumps, fetid canals, or waterlogged marshes.

This pattern has been repeated, with many variations, in almost all regions of the developing world. In Latin America, the problem has been exacerbated by extreme inequalities of land ownership. In many parts of Asia, the difficulties are compounded by some of the highest population densities in the developing world. In Africa, with generally less inequality and fewer people per hectare, the richest lands are often dominated by export agriculture, while the lands of the poor majority are usually of lesser quality, receive less investment, and are more susceptible to drought and desertification.

The common result of these diverse patterns has been the drawing of the poorest into a cycle by which poverty forces growing numbers of people into environmentally vulnerable areas and the resulting environmental stress becomes yet another cause of their continued poverty – a synergism which is today becoming one of the most visible aspects of the PPE crisis. It is no coincidence, for example, that the poorest one quarter of sub-Saharan Africa's population is concentrated on those areas which have been deforested, or overgrazed, or farmed in ways that the soils could not withstand.[58]

The stress on women

By these processes, soils are being eroded, hillsides denuded, and livelihoods washed away along the length of the Himalayan foothills, on the slopes

Poverty has become concentrated in environmentally vulnerable areas - marginal agricultural lands and urban slums.

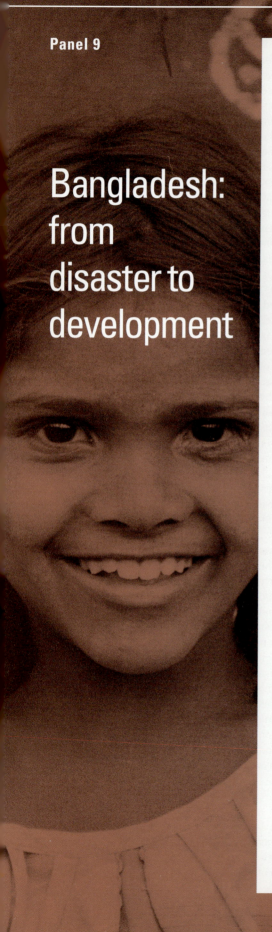

Bangladesh: from disaster to development

When Bangladesh was born in 1971 amid war, flood and famine, many foreign analysts considered it to be a 'basket case' nation with little hope of any future save that of deepening poverty and despair. Today, Bangladesh is more likely to be cited as an example of a very poor country that is making steady progress in the face of great difficulties.

Located in one of the world's most disaster-prone natural environments, Bangladesh exhibits many of the worst symptoms of poverty. For every 1,000 children born, 127 die before their fifth birthday. Two thirds of its under-fives are malnourished. Disease strikes frequently. Disability rates are high. Less than half of Bangladeshi children complete even five years of primary school. And although child labour is outlawed, a quarter of all children work for a living, including six-year-olds who earn pennies a day breaking bricks in the slums.

Yet this grim portrait is slowly being redrawn. Per capita incomes have grown by almost 2% a year over the last decade. Democratic institutions are steadily being strengthened. The nation's fourth five-year development plan incorporates most of the goals adopted at the World Summit for Children. And in 1990, Bangladesh became one of the first nations to ratify the Convention on the Rights of the Child.

Progress has followed promises. After 20 years of hard work, 80% of rural residents are now within 150 metres of a source of safe drinking water – a feat unmatched by many richer nations. Basic health care is also being strengthened. In 1985 less than 2% of Bangladeshi children were immunized against measles – one of the lowest rates in the world. Six years later, the proportion had risen to over 50%.

In 1989, realizing that iodine deficiency disorders (IDD) were widespread, Bangladesh decreed that all edible salt be iodized. A national IDD control programme is now fully operational and that target is expected to be met by early 1994.

Government health services have reached into almost every village – often by relying on ordinary people who offer their homes as monthly outreach sites. This network now promotes basic health interventions such as oral rehydration therapy for diarrhoea and vitamin A supplements to combat blindness.

Bangladesh has also surprised many observers by the progress it has made in family planning. The contraceptive prevalence rate has risen from 3% in 1970 to 30% in 1991, and the country's total fertility rate has fallen from almost 7 births per woman to 4.8, in only two decades.

In addition to government efforts, Bangladesh is also home to several thousand non-governmental organizations – some of which have become internationally renowned for new approaches and for the unprecedented scale and ambition of their operations.

The Grameen Bank began in 1976 as an experiment with a radical idea – that poor people supplied with working capital could generate productive self-employment without external assistance. Now it is the country's fourth largest bank, making small loans to more than 1 million who were previously considered 'unbankable'. Over 80% of clients are women, and the repayment rate is 98%.

The Bangladesh Rural Advancement Committee (BRAC) has grown into one of the world's largest non-governmental organizations, like Grameen winning international acclaim. Emphasizing self-reliance, BRAC organizes thousands of the poorest citizens into community organizations and runs some 15,000 village-based, non-formal schools. Some 70% of its 450,000 students are girls. BRAC earns one third of its income from investments in commercial projects and in-house enterprises. □

of the Andes, in the environmental disaster areas of Haiti and the Dominican Republic, throughout the central highlands of Central America, and in the highlands of Ethiopia where over half of all agricultural land is now significantly eroded.[59] In total, the World Food Council has estimated that there are now perhaps half a billion people who are living and farming on hillsides that are subject to serious erosion of soils.[60] Every year, nearly 17 million more hectares of tropical forests are destroyed; every year, approximately 6 million hectares of dry lands turn into deserts; every year, billions of tons of soil are washed or blown away from lands on which increasing numbers of people who have nowhere else to go must grow their food and earn their living.[61]

In the cities, environmental vulnerability is also taking its toll on the poorest. In addition to the dangers of disease born of overcrowding and the lack of safe water and sanitation, the poor are increasingly subject to unnatural disasters – from the Bhopal chemical leak in India to the explosion of the Cubātao gas pipeline in Brazil. And it is again no coincidence that these disasters claim most of their victims among the shanty communities that have grown up around such facilities because there is nowhere else to go.

In almost all cases, this spiral of poverty and environmental stress bears down with particular weight on the female members of poor communities: they are the ones who have to work even harder to meet the minimum needs of their families when wood for fuel must be fetched from ever greater distances, when water supplies are unreliable and dangerous, and when the degradation of soils means that more work is required to produce less food.

The poverty spiral

Under the impact of these forces that make up the PPE problem, the nature of poverty is in one fundamental respect going through a transformation in many parts of the developing world. Instead of being relatively evenly dispersed geographically, the poor are becoming increasingly concentrated in environmentally marginal and vulnerable areas where they have little choice but to over-exploit already fragile conditions, depleting their resource base still further and condemning themselves and their children to continued poverty (figs. 11, 12, 13, and 14).

PPE problems therefore constitute a vicious circle by which poverty helps to maintain high rates of population growth and increases environmental stress, both of which contribute in their turn to the perpetuation of poverty. And it is a circle from which the poor do not usually have the resources or the opportunities to break free.

It has long been recognized that what is required to break out of this cycle is 'growth from below',[62] brought about by a combination of land reform and labour-intensive employment strategies, credit schemes, training opportunities, the right kind of technologies, and investments in health and education. In addition, millions of poor people today need investments to help them maintain the stability and productivity of soils.

At present, these means of breaking out of the PPE spiral are not available to large numbers of people. In part, the fault lies with governments that have given too little priority to the needs of the poorest. But in part, also, the task of breaking out of the spiral is made more difficult by the industrialized world's policies on aid, debt, trade, and finance which restrict the growth of employment opportunities. Diversification of the economies of the developing countries is essential if the poverty spiral is to be broken, but as the Brundtland Commission concluded in its 1987 report *Our common future*: "*Diversification in ways that will alleviate both poverty and ecological stress is hampered by disadvantageous terms of technology transfer, by protectionism, and by declining financial flows to those countries that most need international finance.*"[63]

Fig. 11 The vulnerable

Number and proportion of the poorest rural people in the developing world who live in areas with low agricultural potential threatened by environmental deterioration.

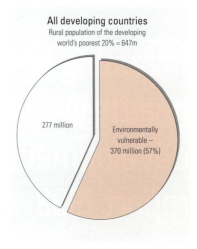

All developing countries
Rural population of the developing world's poorest 20% = 647m

277 million

Environmentally vulnerable – 370 million (57%)

Source: *Adapted from* Environment and the poor: development strategies for a common agenda, *Overseas Development Council, Washington, D.C., 1989.*

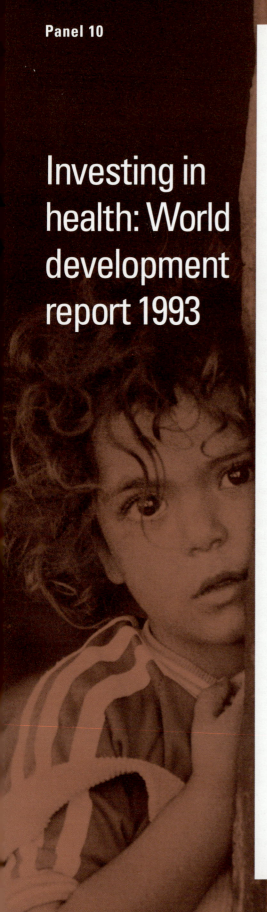

Investing in health: World development report 1993

Throughout the last decade, UNICEF has drawn attention to the fact that major gains in health could be made by the widespread use of a limited number of specific, low-cost health interventions. This year, the annual *World development report* from the World Bank also addresses this issue. The 1993 report aims "*to assist policy makers in realizing the enormous potential returns from their countries' investments in health.*" Its premise is that "*Tools and methods for combating and eliminating much of the remaining burden of disease are now affordable even by the poorest countries.*"

"*In most of the world,*" says the report, "*a great deal of additional health could be obtained from a relatively small number of cost-effective interventions which could be delivered at modest cost and with little need for high-level facilities or medical specialities.*" In the area of child health, the report singles out immunization, plus vitamin A and iodine supplements, as "*a cluster of interventions … that would have the highest cost-effectiveness of any health service available in the world today.*"

As a way of measuring cost-effectiveness, the World Bank report employs a new method of quantifying ill health. First, the number of years of life lost to disease is calculated by subtracting the actual age at death from the expectation of life at that age in a low-mortality population. The impact of disabilities is then calculated by multiplying the expected duration of the disability with a 'severity factor' of up to 0.6 – effectively comparing the disability with loss of life and allowing the two to be added together. Once combined, the losses from death and disability are then adjusted by attaching a variable value to each year lost depending on age. This weighting, arrived at by 'consensus judgement', rises steeply from zero at birth to a peak at age 25, after which it declines steadily with increasing age.

The result is a number which represents disability-adjusted life years or 'DALYs'. The total number of DALYs is a rough measure of the global burden of disease. In total, the Bank calculates that the world lost 1.36 billion DALYs to ill health in 1990. One quarter of this was accounted for by the major childhood diseases.

The number of lost DALYs that can be prevented by a particular health intervention is then used as a measure of cost-effectiveness.

If this method were to be used to determine the priorities of national health programmes worldwide, then the pattern of health spending in the world would look very different. Even taking into account real-world pressures, the Bank says that "*Governments in developing countries should spend far less – on average, about 50% less – than they now do on less cost-effective interventions and instead double or triple spending on basic public health programmes such as immunization and AIDS prevention and on essential clinical services.*"

In particular, the report advocates a "*minimum package of essential clinical services*" consisting of the most basic and cost-effective health interventions. "*Tertiary care and less cost-effective services will continue,*" says the report, "*but public subsidies to them, if they mainly benefit the wealthy, should be phased out during a transitional period.*"

"*Government spending accounts for half of the $168 billion annual expenditures on health in developing countries,*" concludes World Bank President Lewis Preston. "*Too much of this sum goes to specialized care in tertiary facilities that provides little gain for the money spent. Too little goes to low-cost, highly effective programmes such as control and treatment of infectious diseases and of malnutrition.*" □

World development report 1993: Investing in health, World Bank, Washington, D.C., 1993.

Consequences

The continuation of the PPE problem into the 21st century will have consequences extending far beyond its already harsh effects on the poorest billion of the world's people. It is therefore a matter of fundamental self-interest, as well as of altruistic concern, that the rest of the world should accord this problem a new priority.

First of all, the environmental impact of the PPE problem poses a serious threat to large numbers of not-so-poor people who live and work in more prosperous agricultural areas of the developing world. Water flowing across denuded slopes and deforested hillsides erodes exposed soils, carrying them down to the intensively cultivated valley floors, flood plains, and river estuaries; as these sediments are deposited, river levels rise and dams and irrigation works become silted up, wiping out investments and increasing the frequency and severity of floods. According to some estimates, these processes are already threatening the livelihoods of 400 million families who farm the more fertile agricultural areas of the developing world.[64]

Secondly, the increasing pressure on marginal lands, and especially on tropical forests, poses a threat to all – including the populations of the industrialized world – through its well-publicized contribution to the increase in greenhouse gases and to the rapid and accelerating loss of biological diversity. These issues were widely publicized during the United Nations Conference on Environment and Development, held in Rio de Janeiro in 1992, and are clearly set out in Agenda 21, the document that was approved by the world's political leaders at the conclusion of the 'Earth Summit'. They are therefore only mentioned here as a further mechanism by which PPE problems reach out far beyond that one fifth of the world's population that is most directly affected.

Instability

In addition to their worldwide environmental impact, PPE problems are also beginning to transmit international shock waves through their impact on the political stability of the developing nations, with all the costs and risks that such instabilities will pose.

The first casualty is likely to be the progress being made towards representative democracy and the rule of law. The hopes of millions of people have been raised in the scores of countries which have made or are attempting to make the transition from authoritarian rule. Frustration of those hopes by PPE problems will increase economic desperation, leading to further internal migrations, social division, political turmoil, and violent conflicts. In short, there is a clear risk of creating a climate for the return of the dictators and demagogues who have inflicted so much damage on the prospects of so many developing nations in the recent past. This is the danger foreseen by, among others, Adebayo Adedeji, former Executive Secretary of the Economic Commission for Africa, who has said that *"Democracy cannot thrive in conditions of abject poverty,"* or by Dr. Kofi Awoonor, Ghana's Ambassador to the United Nations, who has said that *"Poverty is the father of dictatorship. It is naive to believe that by merely institutionalizing multiparty pluralism and proclaiming free-market systems, a poor country which does not receive adequate returns for its exports, is denied access to technology under intelligent concessionary terms, is overburdened by a crippling debt syndrome, or is virtually a charity case as it battles with the crushing impact of grim social disabilities, will survive as a democracy."*[65]

If these pessimistic scenarios materialize, then another downward spiral would also be set in motion: capital would flow abroad; foreign and domestic investment levels would fall, as would revenues from such stability-dependent sources as tourism; social services such as health and education would be disrupted; less attention would be paid to poverty and environmental degradation; and national resources would once more tend to be diverted to the military, to repression,

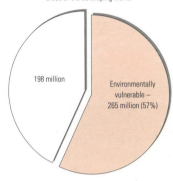

Fig. 13 The vulnerable in Africa

Number and proportion of the poorest rural people in sub-Saharan Africa who live in areas with low agricultural potential threatened by environmental deterioration.

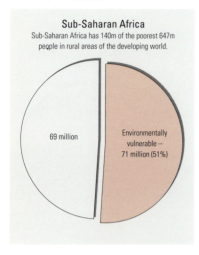

Sub-Saharan Africa

Sub-Saharan Africa has 140m of the poorest 647m people in rural areas of the developing world.

69 million

Environmentally vulnerable – 71 million (51%)

Source: *Adapted from* Environment and the poor: development strategies for a common agenda, *Overseas Development Council, Washington, D.C., 1989.*

and to coping with the consequences of conflict and internal migrations.

In this way, one of the most powerful synergisms of all may be perpetuated – that between instability and poverty. The briefest survey of those places in the world where poverty is at its most severe, and where progress has brought fewest benefits, shows that they are by and large the places which have suffered from prolonged periods of instability, conflict, and repression. In his 1992 statement *An agenda for peace*, the Secretary-General of the United Nations, Boutros Boutros-Ghali, has said that the deepest causes of conflict are "*economic despair, social injustice, and political oppression*". And in its turn, conflict is also one of the most common and devastating causes of poverty and despair.

At the heart of this most destructive of synergisms is the threat to democracy itself: "*Only a society of democratically protected human rights,*" continues *An agenda for peace*, "*can offer the stability that can sustain development over time.*"[66]

The industrialized world

The interaction between PPE problems and national instabilities and conflicts also has obvious repercussions for peace and stability at the international level. In some cases, international action will be required to help protect populations in extreme emergencies, or in failed states where all order has broken down. In other cases, international involvement will be the response to aggression from dictatorial regimes that have come to power by exploiting the frustrations of the poor. The costs and risks of coping with such emergencies, already considerable, are likely to rise substantially in the years ahead. As one distinguished modern historian has written: "*The record indicates that among the possible consequences of rapid population growth, social turbulence and territorial expansion are as plausible as any.*"[67]

Secondly, the PPE problem will also surface in the form of increased migratory pressures as people attempt,

legally or illegally, to escape from lands of no hope to lands of even limited opportunity. Already, an estimated 100 million people are living outside the country in which they were born.[68] According to the United Nations Population Fund (UNFPA), the overwhelming majority of these are economic migrants; at least 20 million are also fleeing from violence, drought, and environmental destruction.[69] As these numbers mount, and as the industrialized countries begin to feel more of the pressure, the connection with the need for a new and poverty-oriented international development effort will become more and more evident.

Lastly, poverty and desperation are also known to travel across international borders in the ugly disguises of terrorism and the traffic in drugs.

The prosperity problem

PPE problems, however large and complex, are only one element of the crisis that is gathering over the 21st century. The other major component of that crisis arises from a different direction – the effects of rising prosperity.

It has already been mentioned that the present threat to the biosphere comes overwhelmingly from the established industrial nations. According to some estimates, for example, the impact of the average American citizen on the global environment is approximately 3 times that of the average Italian, 13 times that of the average Brazilian, 35 times that of the average Indian, 140 times that of the average Bangladeshi, and more than 250 times that of a citizen born into one of the least developed nations of sub-Saharan Africa.[70] This again is an issue which has been widely discussed elsewhere.[71]

Less widely discussed are the likely consequences if far more populous countries in the world successfully pursue a similar pattern of progress.

Many of the largest nations on earth, particularly in Asia, have reasonable expectations of economic growth in the years ahead. Given the global reach of television and video, and their dynamic effects on human aspirations and lifestyles, it appears likely that many of these populous and soon-to-be-more-prosperous nations of the world will aspire to, and in many cases begin to achieve, the same kind of material progress that prevails today in the established industrial countries.

Who would deny that this is their right? Yet who would deny that this right cannot be realized without pushing environmental tolerance beyond its limits? Clearly, the industrialized world is in no position to wave an environmental warning flag at any nation in the developing world or suggest that it should not aspire to higher levels of material progress; nothing could be more unrealistic than expecting millions of people to continue travelling by bullock cart and washing their clothes in streams and rivers before settling down to watch reruns of 'Dallas' and 'Dynasty'.

Yet just to bring energy consumption in the developing world up to the level of the industrialized world today, for example, would increase total world energy consumption at least fivefold. And as the Brundtland Commission has reported, "*The planetary ecosystem could not stand this, especially if the increases were based on non-renewable fossil fuels. Threats of global warming and acidification of the environment most probably rule out even a doubling of energy use based on present mixes of primary sources.*"[72]

China's present rate of economic progress, for example, would, in one generation, mean a level of economic development similar to that of the Republic of Korea today. At that point, China's economy would be the largest in the world, its impact on the environment would be similar to that of the United States, and its carbon dioxide emissions would exceed those of all today's industrialized nations put together.[73]

Similar examples could be derived from India, whose population will surpass that of China early in the 21st century and whose middle classes, many with aspirations to lifestyles similar to those in industrialized countries, already number at least 100 million, a population greater than that of any Western European country.

No alternative

This dilemma is clearly the great catch-22 of the 21st century. For poor countries to remain within the PPE spiral already discussed is to invite disaster. But for four fifths of the world's people to follow the path of development blazed by the one fifth who live in today's industrialized nations is to invite a disaster of a different kind.

Freezing the status quo is not an option either in principle or in practice. As the authors of *Beyond the limits* have pointed out, 20 years after their original publication *Limits to growth*, "*A sustainable society would not freeze into permanence the current inequitable patterns of distribution. It would certainly not permit the persistence of poverty. To do so would not be sustainable for two reasons. First, the poor would not and should not stand for it. Second, keeping any part of the population in poverty would not, except under dire coercive measures, allow the population to stabilize.*"[74]

The only way forward, however difficult it may be to find, is a cooperative international effort to achieve three principal objectives:

☐ Resolving PPE problems by bringing to an end the worst aspects of poverty, slowing population growth, and investing in the rural and urban environments within which today's poor live and work;[75]

☐ Making the transition to new paths of progress in the industrialized countries in order to maintain or improve the quality of life while significantly reducing environmental impact. One criterion of such a new definition of progress would be 'can the developing countries, if they so choose, aspire to similar lifestyles without exceeding the planet's capacity?';

☐ Assisting all developing countries to develop the kind of economies and technologies which will allow them to pursue their chosen path of material development without overstepping local and global environmental limits.

These objectives are expressed

Fig. 14 The vulnerable in Latin America
Number and proportion of the poorest rural people in Latin America who live in areas with low agricultural potential threatened by environmental deterioration.

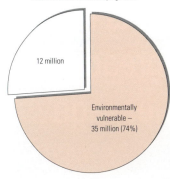

Latin America
Latin America has 47m of the poorest 647m people in rural areas of the developing world.

12 million

Environmentally vulnerable – 35 million (74%)

Source: *Adapted from* Environment and the poor: development strategies for a common agenda, *Overseas Development Council, Washington, D.C., 1989.*

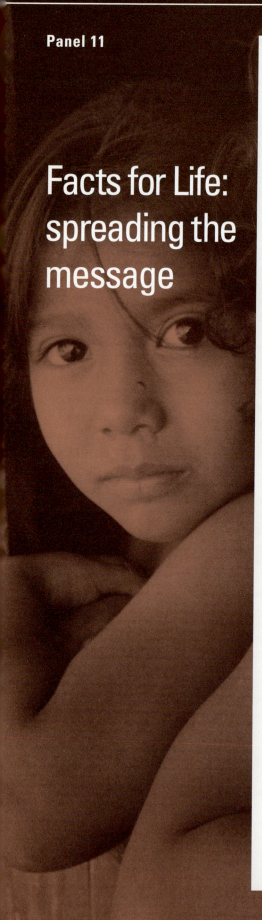

Facts for Life: spreading the message

June 1993 saw the launch of the second edition of *Facts for Life* – the book which brings together today's scientific consensus on practical, low-cost ways of protecting the lives and the normal growth of children.

Since it first appeared in 1989, more than 9 million copies of the first edition of *Facts for Life* have been published and the text has been translated into 176 languages. The second edition, carrying a new chapter on early childhood development, is co-published by four United Nations agencies – UNICEF, WHO, UNESCO and UNFPA. Over 160 international non-governmental organizations are partners in the venture. The second edition takes into account the many comments received from users over the last four years.

Facts for Life's basic messages are organized into chapters on timing births, safe motherhood, breastfeeding, child growth, immunization, diarrhoeal disease, respiratory infections, hygiene, malaria, AIDS, and child development. But in many of the more than 100 countries where the book has been translated or adapted, its messages have been tailored to fit specific national or local needs. Chapters have been added or substituted, usually with the help of leading national experts, on subjects ranging from smoking and drug abuse to dental hygiene, accidents, and sexually transmitted diseases.

The *Facts for Life* book cannot reach more than a small fraction of the families who might benefit from its messages. It is therefore aimed at all those who are in a position to reach out to a wide public – community health workers, teachers, mass media, religious organizations, voluntary agencies, the business community, and the government agencies. The response from all of these potential communicators has given *Facts for Life* an unprecedented outreach in the last four years.

In addition to being used by the health services of most nations, *Facts for Life* has become part of the formal school curriculum and/or adult literacy programmes in more than 30 nations. In Mexico, almost a million copies have been printed for use as school textbooks. In China, 1 million copies have been published in 12 languages. In Iran, *Facts for Life* has been adapted for the national literacy campaign, reaching 2 million people, mainly women. In Myanmar, 200,000 copies of the national version have been produced for schools, health centres, water and sanitation workers, and religious organizations. In Nigeria, 300,000 copies have been produced in four major languages for schools, nursing colleges and religious leaders.

In most countries, the media have responded with television and radio spots, serializations of *Facts for Life* messages, and the inclusion of messages in hundreds of soap operas and popular radio programmes. In Brazil, a major supermarket chain has put *Facts for Life* messages on 120 million plastic bags. In Kenya, 10 million matchboxes carry the messages. In Turkey, they have appeared on 2 million milk cartons.

New knowledge can only ever be one factor among the many forces that decide health behaviour. Poverty and social pressures, education and confidence, have a powerful effect on the choices people have and the decisions they take. But all families have a right to today's practical, scientific information which could help them to protect the lives and the health of their children by methods they can act on *now* and at a cost they can afford today. □

The second edition of *Facts for Life* is available from, UNICEF House, DH40, Facts for Life Unit, 3 UN Plaza, New York, NY 10017, USA, or through local UNICEF offices. A companion booklet – *Using Facts for Life* – will also be available from late 1993.

here as generalities – masking a million practical difficulties. But the longer the beginning of that transition is postponed, the greater the difficulties will be. The geopolitical changes of the last four years have opened up a dramatic and unforeseen opportunity to make that beginning. As the United Nations Under-Secretary-General for Humanitarian Affairs, Jan Eliasson, said at the end of 1992, *"If at this stage of history, with the ending of the cold war and the beginning of a new era, we cannot put the welfare of human beings at the centre of all our concerns and operations, and really prove that the whole idea of organizing ourselves in societies and international organizations was to improve the conditions in which we all live, then we are failing humanity."*[76]

New concepts of security

An essential element of this change is a redefinition of what is meant by security. Following the debate caused by the publication of his book *The rise and fall of the great powers*, historian Paul Kennedy has attempted the difficult task of applying some of its lessons to the task of preparing for the 21st century. *"Governments and peoples,"* he writes, *"need to reconsider their older definitions of what constitutes a threat to national and international security. Regardless of whether the cold war is over or whether an end can be brought to Middle East rivalries, there now exist vast non-military threats to the safety and well-being of the peoples of this planet which deserve attention... Just as nation-state rivalries are being overtaken by bigger issues, we may have to think about the future on a far broader scale than has characterized thinking about international politics in the past."*[77]

In many developing nations, and particularly in sub-Saharan Africa, it is already clear that national security is threatened by PPE problems, including environmental degradation on a scale that no invading army could contemplate. Yet most societies are still devoting many times more resources to military capacity than to environmental protection.

In the industrialized countries, also, threats to national security are now far more likely to arise from environmental disputes, cross-border pollution by acid rains, or uncontrollable migratory pressures, than from any military offensive. Internationally, the greatest threats to stability are likely to arise from the collapse of democracies, and of social order and cohesion, as a result of mounting PPE problems.[78] Globally, the threat to the biosphere from unrestrained pursuit of present patterns of progress is, as many observers have pointed out, *"every bit as unthinkable as the consequences of unrestrained nuclear war"*.[79]

These new threats to national and international security clearly call for new responses. In particular, it is essential that the most powerful nation in today's world should use its immense influence in the cause of managing the great transition to a sustainable future. And in the United States today, voices are beginning to be raised in support of the idea that policies should be radically reoriented in response to PPE problems. Among the most thoughtful of those voices, two may be excerpted here:

☐ *"I am afraid that twenty years from now, when they write the history of the twentieth century, they will say that the most surprising event was that following the collapse of the Eastern bloc, the world's major power, the United States, did not move with vision and decisiveness to help institute a new and fair world order aimed at preventing aggression, reallocating resources from militarization to human self-improvement at home and abroad, and pursuing a development path globally that the biofilm can withstand."*[80]

☐ *"Improbable or not, something like the Marshall Plan – a Global Marshall Plan, if you will – is now urgently needed. The scope and complexity of this plan will far exceed those of the original; what is required now is a plan that combines large-scale, long-term, carefully targeted financial aid to developing nations, massive efforts to design and then transfer to poor nations the new technologies needed for sustainable economic progress, a*

In many developing nations, national security is threatened by environmental degradation on a scale that no invading army could contemplate.

world-wide program to stabilize world population, and binding commitments by the industrial nations to accelerate their own transition to an environmentally responsible pattern of life."[81]

Although these voices might be regarded as idealistic, they are not crying from as far out in the political wilderness as one might think. The first of the opinions quoted above is that of Peter C. Goldmark, President of the Rockefeller Foundation, and the second is taken from the writings of Senator Al Gore, now Vice-President of the United States.

The first test

The PPE problem, the environmental threat from present patterns of progress, and the need to make the great transition to a sustainable future, set the broad context for any attempt to bring the basic benefits of progress to all communities and meet the great human goals discussed in the first part of this report.

To meet these challenges, national action and international cooperation are needed in many different fields – in the rules and practices of international trade, in more people-oriented and labour-intensive national development policies, in restoring financial flows and investments to the developing world, in the negotiation of environmental agreements, and in scientific cooperation and the transfer of technology.

But in relation to PPE problems, in particular, it is clearly now possible to make a major impact by renewing efforts to overcome the worst aspects of the poverty that provides much of the impetus for both population growth and environmental stress in the developing world. Reducing child deaths, controlling malnutrition and disease, increasing family food production, and making family planning available to all are ways of jump-starting a solution to many of these seemingly intractable problems. And achieving the basic human goals that have been agreed by the majority of the world's political leaders could therefore be considered a first test of the international community's willingness and capacity to begin making the great transition.

The final part of this report therefore looks in more detail at the central contribution which the achievement of basic human goals could make to the resolution of PPE problems – to the meeting of minimum human needs, to the stabilization of populations, and to the easing of environmental pressures.

The synergism of solutions

Part 1 of this report summarized the progress and the potential in several major and specific areas of child well-being. Its conclusion was that the relevant knowledge, technology, and outreach capacity have been developed to the point at which some of the most basic benefits of progress could now be put at the disposal of all families in almost all countries and at a modest cost. In particular, national governments and the international community are now in a position, should they so decide, to bring about and sustain very significant improvements in the survival, health, nutrition, and education of many millions of the world's children. Specific goals which reflect this potential have been agreed by the political leaders of most nations.

Part 2 has mapped the broader landscape in which this potential advance must take place, drawing attention to the mutually reinforcing negative effects of continued poverty, rapid population growth, and increasing environmental stress – the PPE problem which threatens to overwhelm not only present potential but also past gains.

Part 3 looks at the relationship between potential and threat, and examines how the achieving of the basic human goals could make a fundamental contribution to resolving the problems that loom as the 21st century approaches.

To recap, those goals include:
- Control of the major childhood diseases;
- A halving of child malnutrition;
- A one-third reduction in under-five death rates;
- A halving of maternal mortality rates;
- The provision of safe water to all communities;
- A basic education for all children;
- The universal availability of family planning information and services.

Each of these goals is directly related to the defusing of the PPE problem. But in order to examine these relationships, it will be convenient to group the areas of potential progress into three: health and nutrition; education; and family planning.

HEALTH AND NUTRITION

Reaching basic human health goals would strike at one of the main roots of the PPE problem.

First, improved health is one of the most powerful of all weapons for attacking poverty. Whether judged by the economic losses caused by specific diseases[82] or by the economic returns earned by investments in water supply,[83] the overwhelming testimony of recent years is that advances in health and nutrition help to improve productivity and to increase the returns on other forms of investment.

In the short term, it is obvious that frequent illness drains time, energy, and resources from the business of earning a living, causing loss of working days in fields, factories, and homes, and a further loss of adult time and energy in looking after sick children. In addition, the direct costs of medical expenses claim, on average, about 10% of family income in the world's poor communities.

In the longer term, there is an obvious and profound connection between the mental and physical development of children and the social and economic development of their societies.

The first contribution that would be made by reaching basic health goals would therefore be to enhance both the short-term and long-term economic prospects of poor communities.

There is an obvious and profound connection between the mental and physical development of children and the social and economic development of their societies.

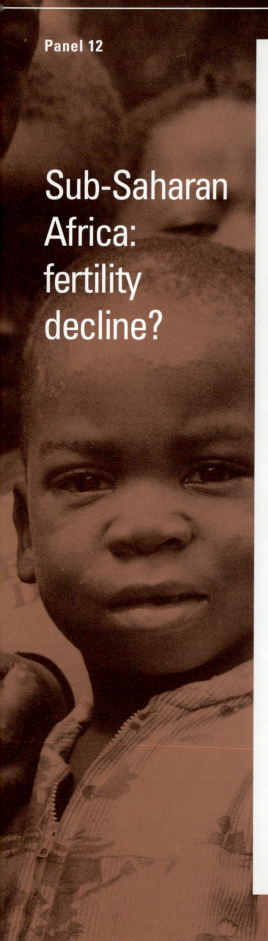

Sub-Saharan Africa: fertility decline?

Sub-Saharan Africa is the only region of the developing world that has not yet undergone a widespread decline in fertility. Some demographers believe that a decline has now begun; others are not yet prepared to commit themselves, arguing that the evidence is mixed.

Demographic and Health Surveys (DHS) have recently been conducted in 21 sub-Saharan African nations. Reports from 13 such studies have been published, and preliminary results are available for four more.

The studies, in conjunction with other evidence, make it clear that fertility has begun to decline in at least three of the countries studied — Botswana, Kenya, and Zimbabwe.

Even for these nations, statistics on fertility change, over time, are far from satisfactory. But other observed trends lend weight to the finding that there has been a decline in the total fertility rate (TFR) of more than one birth per woman. The reported rate of modern contraceptive use, for example, has risen significantly: in Zimbabwe, 43% of married women now use a modern method of family planning; in Botswana the figure is 33%, and in Kenya 27%.

More confirmation comes from surveys asking women how many children they want. In Kenya, the answer fell very sharply from an average of 5.8 in 1984 to 4.4 in 1989. Among women aged 40-44, the ideal number of children averaged 5.5; among those aged 15-19 the average answer given was 3.7.

Botswana, Kenya and Zimbabwe have also fared better than many African nations in all four of the areas of progress most commonly associated with falling fertility — rising female education, falling child mortality, well-run family planning programmes, and a degree of economic progress.

The most dramatic decline has occurred in Zimbabwe where DHS results suggest that the TFR has fallen by 1.2 births per woman between 1981-1984 and 1985-1988. Botswana has seen a decline of 0.8 over the same period. In Kenya, the TFR seems to have fallen by 1.5 births per woman in total and by 0.5 between 1987 and 1989, suggesting that the decline in fertility could be accelerating sharply.

It is also possible that fertility has begun to fall in Burundi, Mali, Nigeria, Senegal, and Togo, though in all of these the fall in TFR is less marked and the supporting evidence is less convincing.

In Nigeria — with almost a quarter of sub-Saharan Africa's people — the available statistics suggest a decline in the TFR of 1.3 births per woman from 1982 to 1988. This is the largest measured decline of any country in sub-Saharan Africa to date, but the finding is suspect; it is not consistent, for example, with surveys showing that only 6% of married women in Nigeria use some form of contraception and that only 3.5% use modern methods. Overall, it seems likely that a decline has begun in the more populous areas of the south-west and possibly in the south-east.

Those who argue that no general decline in fertility has yet begun in sub-Saharan Africa point to the fact that traditional values strongly favour large families and that the use of contraception is approximately 20 percentage points lower than could be expected when compared to other countries at similar levels of economic development.

Others argue that the circumstances that determine family size are changing, and that Africans will respond exactly as other populations have done — providing that sufficient priority is given to reducing child deaths, educating women, and making modern family planning methods widely and conveniently available. □

Most of the information in this panel is drawn from Foote, Karen A., and others, eds., *Demographic Change in Sub-Saharen Africa*, National Academy Press, Washington, D.C., 1993

Health and population growth

Secondly, reaching basic health goals would have a long-term effect on population growth.

The present potential for improving children's health and saving children's lives is clearly enormous – so enormous that it has led some to question the wisdom of deploying such techniques as immunization, ORT, and antibiotics, on the grounds that increasing child survival rates will merely exacerbate population problems.

This argument is not only unethical, it is profoundly mistaken.

It is an unethical argument because it implies that an acceptable response to the population problem is to deliberately withhold basic benefits of progress from the poorest quarter of the world's people in order that a significant percentage of their children should continue to die. If such a precept were allowed to prevail, then the struggle towards a civilized and sustainable future would be defeated not by any population explosion or environmental disaster, but by a catastrophe of the human spirit.

And it is a mistaken argument because it is based on a misperception of the relationship between child deaths and population growth. That relationship has many facets, but overall it reflects the empirical fact that a significant and sustained reduction in child deaths is almost invariably a precondition for a rise in contraceptive use and a sustained fall in fertility.[84]

One underlying aspect of that relationship is that the death of a child is often quickly compensated for by a new pregnancy.[85] Even in cases where this is not the conscious intention, the death of an infant means that breastfeeding stops, and with it the contraceptive effect. For both of these reasons, high child death rates usually mean that more children are born.

A second facet of the relationship is that if many children die then parents tend to insure, and often to over-insure, by having a larger number of children than they actually want.[86] More broadly, where confidence in child survival remains low, parents and communities tend not to progress to the stage of building families by conscious planning.[87] Conversely, when child death rates fall and the relationship between the number of births and eventual family size becomes more predictable, family planning becomes a more attractive proposition.

Many studies over the last decade have demonstrated these effects. They have been summed up by the United Nations Population Division in one sentence: *"Improvements in child survival, which increase the predictability of the family building process, trigger the transition from natural to controlled fertility behaviour."*[88]

That conclusion was also endorsed by the 1992 'Earth Summit' in Rio de Janeiro, and by its Secretary-General, Maurice Strong: *"The effort to reduce child illness and malnutrition and to reach the goals of the World Summit for Children is crucial not only for its own sake but also as a means of helping to slow population growth and make possible environmentally sustainable development in the 21st century and beyond."*

Threshold effect

This link between reducing child deaths and reducing fertility levels has now reached a critical point. To see why, it is necessary to look in a little more detail at the different stages of that relationship. As figure 15 shows, the early stages of decline in child deaths often have little effect on fertility. At this stage, a high under-five mortality rate affects the rate of population growth in two contradictory ways: it means, obviously, that fewer children survive to have children of their own and, all other things being equal, this might lower population growth rates by a few percentage points; but it also means that fertility levels remain high, as parents cannot be confident in the survival of their existing children; this tends to have a much more pronounced effect in keeping population growth rates high.

It is at the subsequent stage of this process, when under-five mortality

Fig. 15 Child deaths and births

Changes in the total fertility rate (average number of births per woman) compared with changes in under-five mortality rates. For each region, the points on the graph show the situation in 1960, 1970, 1980, and 1990.

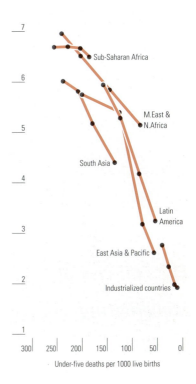

The total fertility rate is the number of children that would be born to a woman who lives to the end of her child-bearing years and who bears children at each age in accordance with prevailing age-specific fertility rates.

Sources: *United Nations*, World population prospects: the 1992 revision, *1993; and UNICEF, unpublished data.*

The real risk of exacerbating population problems comes not from efforts to bring such benefits as immunization and antibiotics to all the world's children: it comes from the failure to do so.

rates begin to fall from around 150 per 1,000 live births to 100 per 1,000 and then to 50 per 1,000, that contraceptive use tends to rise more sharply and fertility to fall more steeply. Figure 16, for example, shows that in 108 countries for which the figures are available, contraceptive use rates remain below 20% in those countries where under-five mortality remains above 150 per 1,000. Only when child deaths fall below 100 per 1,000 does contraceptive use rise to 50% or more.[89] Similarly, figure 15 shows that where under-five mortality rates remain high, the fertility rate tends to remain at six, seven, or eight births per woman. It is when child deaths fall steeply that fertility declines to four, three, or two births per woman.

The significance of this pattern, for the population dimension of the PPE problem, is that many countries of the developing world have already passed through the early stages of this process and are poised on the threshold of what could and should be a period of rapid fertility decline; entering that stage depends on a continuing decline in under-five mortality.

This historical pattern is likely to become even more pronounced because, today, almost all countries have well-established, if not always adequately funded, family planning programmes. Further gains in child health and survival can therefore be translated, more quickly than in the past, into reductions in fertility.

In sum, doing what can now be done to improve child health and reduce child deaths would not only be a significant advance in its own right, it would also be an important contribution to the lowering of birth rates. Conversely, to allow progress to slacken now would be to risk leaving many developing countries on the threshold of substantial falls in fertility without actually taking the plunge.

In other words, the real risk of exacerbating population problems today does not come from efforts to bring such benefits as immunization and antibiotics to all the world's children: it comes from the failure to do so.

EDUCATION

The goals that have been established for the end of this century include providing primary school education for at least 80% of children – both boys and girls – by the year 2000.

After three decades of impressive progress, primary school enrolment and retention rates have stagnated or fallen in many African and some Latin American countries in the 1980s. On present trends, therefore, the target of primary school education for at least 80% will be one of the most difficult goals to achieve. But without progress towards that goal, it will become increasingly difficult to cope with the PPE challenge.

The links between educational advance and resolving PPE problems are many. To begin with, education, like health, helps to loosen the hold of poverty. Many studies, particularly those initiated by the World Bank in recent years, have demonstrated this effect. In agriculture, for example, studies in Malaysia, the Republic of Korea, and Thailand, and more recently in Bangladesh, India, Nepal, Pakistan, and several Latin American countries, have shown that farmers with schooling are more productive than similarly situated farmers without education.[90] Overall, increases in literacy levels and in primary school enrolment have been found to be strongly associated with more rapid increases in per capita incomes and with greater economic equality.[91] Other studies have shown that the economic returns from investments in primary education exceed those of any other kind of investment.

Such conclusions confirm what common sense suggests – that better-educated people can participate more fully in the processes of modernization and development, and are better able to raise their own incomes and contribute to the economic development of their nations.

Education and environment

Secondly, achieving the goal of a basic education for all is one of the most fundamental prerequisites for managing the environmental dimension of the PPE problem.

Preventing further deterioration of the vulnerable environments in which the world's poorest people are increasingly concentrated will require a wide range of interventions. It will require, for example, trade liberalization and increased financial flows to help diversify employment opportunities. It will also require investment in new methods of farming, and especially in techniques of soil and water management, to enable the millions who remain in agriculture to meet their needs in sustainable ways. The years ahead will therefore see a rising need for training and retraining; for the dissemination of new scientific knowledge; for the introduction of new varieties of plants and new ways of farming; for the promotion of knowledge about environmental dangers to health; for a widening public sensitivity to the vulnerability and interdependence of ecosystems; and for an increase in awareness of the choices, alternatives, and long-term consequences of the many decisions that must constantly be made as societies become more complex. Environmentally sound methods of farming, in particular, are very much more knowledge-intensive than most conventional methods.[92]

All of these changes will be necessary if environmental problems are to be coped with. And all depend heavily on education. Unless the goal of a basic education for all can be reached, millions of people will be denied knowledge, choice, and opportunity, rendering them less able to make informed decisions about their own futures and less prepared to adapt to the many changes that lie ahead.

Education and population

Finally, the spread of education is also of the most basic relevance to the third element of the PPE problem – rapid population growth.

In particular, the education of girls has been shown to be one of the most basic determinants of fertility decline.[93]

Educated women usually have more opportunities, more awareness of family planning possibilities, and are more likely to discuss and decide with their partners how many children to have and when. They are also more likely to marry late, to postpone the first pregnancy, to leave more time between births, and to have fewer children in total.[94]

These effects are particularly strong if education continues for more than just two or three years. In one study, conducted in a cross-section of countries, the average number of children born to women with no secondary education was approximately seven, while for women whose education had progressed to secondary level the average was approximately three – even after factors such as income were taken into account.[95]

Increasingly, this female education factor is coming to be seen as a key to the population issue. Addressing the question of what can be done to defuse the population crisis in the immediate future, the President of the Population Council, Margaret Catley-Carlson, comments: *"The biggest answer is known to us already. Of all the social and economic forms of investment which affect fertility behavior, the level of education of women stands out as the most consistent...*

"In several high-fertility traditional societies, women who have completed primary school and above have about three children less than their unschooled or moderately schooled (1 to 3 years) counterparts. The observed reduction in marital fertility is linked to delayed marriage, effective contraceptive use, and, plausibly, the higher expectations held by educated mothers for their children...

"A girl with secondary education typically marries at 21. A girl with none marries at 17. If the higher age were global, there would be close to 1 billion fewer of us before our planet reached population stability."[96]

Drop-out rates

Over the last three decades, the developing world has made enormous

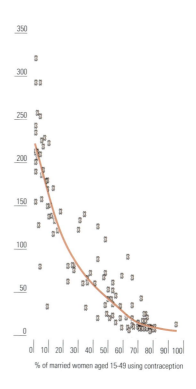

Fig. 16 Confidence in survival
Under-five mortality rates (per 1000 live births) related to levels of contraception in 108 countries of the developing world.

% of married women aged 15-49 using contraception

Sources: *United Nations,* World population prospects: the 1992 revision, *1993; and* UNICEF, *unpublished data.*

43

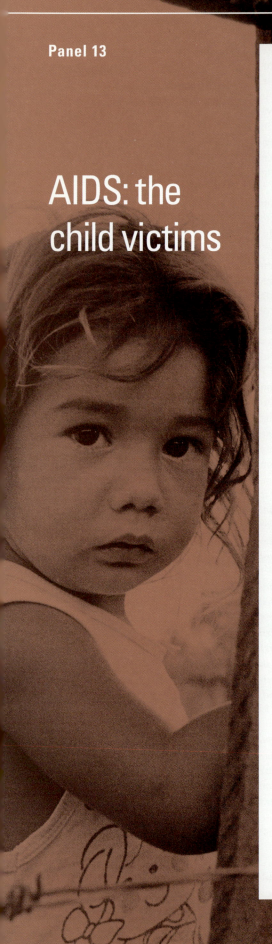

AIDS: the child victims

As the world enters its second decade of fighting the AIDS epidemic, the reports from the front are bleak. In several African countries AIDS is overtaking measles and malaria as a leading killer of children, and hard-won gains in reducing child mortality are being reversed.

In total, the World Health Organization (WHO) estimates that over 13 million people, 1 million of them children, have become infected with HIV. Over 2 million have died.

In sub-Saharan Africa about one adult in 40 is infected with HIV, and in some cities the rate is one in three; in Thailand the rate is 1 in 50. One in four new infections occurs in Asia, and by the end of the decade, if current trends continue, more Asians than Africans will be infected each year. By that time at least 30 million adults and children will be HIV infected: the toll of AIDS deaths may go as high as 1.8 million a year.

Most of these deaths will be in the developing world, and most will be women and children, since the rate of infection in women is rising steeply. A child born to an HIV-infected mother has a 1-in-3 chance of being born with the virus. Such children have an 80% chance of dying by the age of five. Those spared the infection itself are at risk because of their parents' inability to care for them. WHO estimates that there will be 10 million children on their own in Africa by the end of the decade – orphaned, abandoned or runaways, vulnerable in their turn to HIV infection as they take to life on the streets.

By striking people during their most productive years – about two thirds of those infected are under 25 – AIDS is robbing nations as well as families of their able-bodied workers. In Malawi, for example, with one of the world's highest incidences of AIDS, the income lost already amounts to 7% of the nation's gross domestic product, a proportion which is due to double and perhaps even triple by the year 2000. A fifth of the Government's health budget is taken up by AIDS treatment.

The chances of developing an effective vaccine within the decade remain speculative. The best hope lies in prevention, primarily by public health education. In almost all countries, programmes for AIDS prevention are increasingly mobilizing every possible resource for reaching the public. Uganda's programme in sex education and self-esteem for primary school children and their parents has been followed through into secondary schools and colleges; a recent Ministry of Health survey found that over 60% of Ugandans now know how AIDS is spread. Most nations are using a combination of schools programmes and mass media – including television, radio, and popular music and theatre.

Results have been mixed, but there are signs of hope as experience is gained. The use of condoms has risen wherever the public has been informed; in Thailand, for example, condom use has increased from 10 million to 120 million a year. And in countries which have actively focused on sex education for the younger generation, young people are beginning to adopt safer sexual behaviour, including reducing the number of their sexual partners. □

educational strides. Even though total numbers of school-age children doubled between 1960 and 1990, the proportion enrolled in primary school has climbed from under half to more than three quarters.[97]

In total, over 90% of children in the developing world now start school – showing that the institutional capacity and the initial motivation already exist for the achievement of near-universal primary education. But in many countries the poor quality of the education on offer, combined with limited job opportunities and the need for children to help their families in fields and homes, means that large numbers drop out of school before completing even one or two years. In South Asia and South America, for example, more than 95% of children enrol in grade 1 of primary school, but only about 50% reach grade 5 (fig. 17).[98] The greatest educational priority for the 1990s is therefore to ensure that all children not only start school but remain there long enough to acquire literacy, numeracy, and basic attitudes and skills which will help them to improve their circumstances and to cope with the many changes that lie ahead.

At the moment, in spite of formal commitments by governments, it must be said that this task is being given too little priority. In some countries, an acceleration towards education for all is beginning, but in most regions the achievement of this goal looks unlikely. Primary education, the most important investment of all, is at the moment claiming only a small percentage of government budgets in the developing world and only about 2% of all aid for development.

Even if the extra resources can be found, through economic growth, or the restructuring of national budgets, or increases in aid, the task will not be easy. But the experience of several countries over recent years has shown that great gains can be made and sustained at an affordable cost.[99] The principal elements of these successful strategies appear to be: the use of para-teachers in preschools and primary schools; short teacher-training periods; regular support and supervision of teacher performance; small school units close to the communities served; low capital costs of school buildings; active involvement of communities and parents; relevant basic curricula presented in an interesting way; school calendars and timetables that take into account the seasonal demands for children to help in agriculture; and the support of local non-governmental organizations.

The difficulties of finding and carrying through the right mix of strategies to achieve universal primary education in the 1990s are enormous. But so are the consequences of failure. Achieving the goal of a basic education for all children would help to weaken the grip of all of the main protagonists in the PPE spiral – contributing to economic progress for the poor, greater capacity to respond to and deal with environmental problems, and the slower growth and earlier stabilization of populations.

FAMILY PLANNING

The basic human goals for the year 2000 also include the making available of family planning information and services to all who want them – with due respect to each country's cultural, religious, and social traditions.

The importance of this goal for responding to the PPE problem is obvious in that fewer births mean slower population growth and reduced environmental stress. But it is less widely appreciated that family planning can also bring significant improvements in health, survival, nutrition, education, and the quality of life for both mothers and children (figs. 18 and 19). It is therefore one of the most powerful means of breaking into the synergisms of the PPE spiral, and helping to combat the poverty which gives that spiral its impetus.

As with education, the family planning goal should be seen in the context of recent achievement. In only three decades, the proportion of married women in the developing world who are using some form of modern family

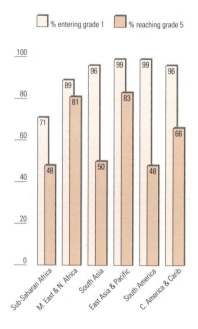

Fig. 17 Primary schooling

Percentages of the developing world's children in the appropriate age range starting primary school and reaching grade 5.

☐ % entering grade 1   ☐ % reaching grade 5

Source: UNICEF calculations from data supplied by UNESCO, mostly for 1988 to 1990.

45

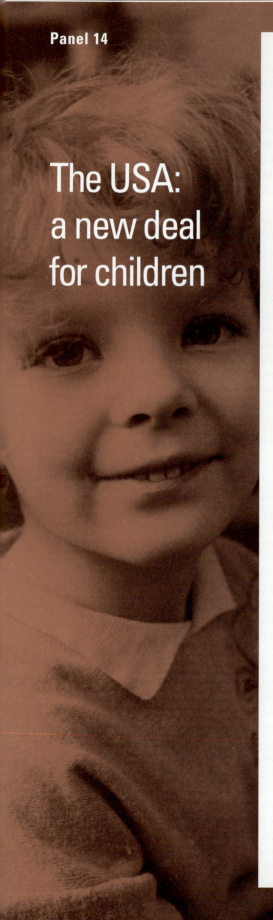

The USA: a new deal for children

An increasing proportion of children in the world's richest nation are in trouble. While America's economy grew by approximately 20% in the 1980s, some 4 million more American children fell into poverty. In total, one in five youngsters now lives below the poverty line – a rate twice that of any other industrialized country.

Other social markers document the decline. Child immunization has fallen as low as 10% in certain inner-city areas; in the western hemisphere only Bolivia and Haiti had lower overall rates. Preventable disease began to rise: more than 55,000 measles cases were reported from 1989 to 1991, including 64 deaths – the highest number in two decades.

Reported child abuse cases also tripled during the 1980s; about three children now die each day of maltreatment. Despite the Government's much-publicized war on drugs, substance abuse and related crime spiralled upwards; an estimated 375,000 drug-exposed infants including 'crack babies' are born each year. Violence stalks streets and schools; 30% of inner-city children have known someone killed by the time they are 15 years old. Today, 31% of the homeless are families with children, up from 21% in the early 1980s.

Some of the changes affecting American children – such as the sharp rise in single parenthood – are beyond the immediate reach of government. But policies to mitigate the effects have generally been inadequate, failing to provide a safety net for children. Welfare programmes were cut back during the 1980s, including the programme for Aid to Families with Dependent Children. More than 1.1 million single-parent families were pushed below the poverty line during the decade.

Racial inequities remain. Infant mortality, for example, is 8 per 1,000 births in white America; black infant mortality is running at 18 per 1,000 – higher than in Cuba or Poland. "*We are in danger of becoming two nations – one of first world privilege and another of third world deprivation,*" warns Marian Wright Edelman, head of the Children's Defense Fund.

Many of the policy objectives of the Clinton Administration, including the President's stated ambition to raise all families with a working parent out of poverty, point to a new deal for American children. Universal health coverage, for example, would bring its greatest benefits to the estimated 8 million children without health care.

The Family and Medical Leave Act, blocked and weakened by the past two Administrations, was quickly signed into law. Although it does not approach the standards of many European countries, it grants up to 12 weeks of unpaid leave to care for newborns or sick relatives and will ease the pressure on many American families.

President Clinton has also declared that immunization is a right for all children – "*like clean water and clean air.*" Congress has allocated increased funding to expand the nation's vaccination programme, and has acted in support of the President's proposal to boost Head Start, one of the most successful child development programmes in US history.

In his address to the United Nations General Assembly in September 1993, the President also spoke of a new commitment to the world's children: "*Just as our own nation has launched new reforms to ensure that every child in America has adequate health care, we must do more to get basic vaccines and other treatments for curable diseases to children around the world. It's the best investment we'll ever make.*" □

planning method has increased from about 10% to about 50%. This is an extraordinary demonstration of the fact that fundamental and large-scale changes in human attitudes and behaviour can be brought about within a relatively short space of years.

"*In the early 1960s,*" write John Rowley and Halfdan Mahler of the International Planned Parenthood Federation, "*fewer than 15 million couples in the developing world outside China were using contraception. Today, some 380 million couples in the developing world are taking charge of their fertility – over half of all couples in the child-bearing years.*

"*There is now no doubt that the world is in transition, social and demographic. We are on the way to creating a world in which mankind's success in reducing death rates is matched by a move towards fewer, healthier, planned births. Such a world will be one in which women everywhere have a right to control their own fertility. It will be one in which reproductive health is a matter of universal care and concern. It will be a world where population growth rates no longer fuel urban and environmental pressures which help perpetuate gross disparities of wealth and poverty and which lead to continuing destruction of the 'spaceship in which we travel'.*"[100]

That transition is not yet complete. Fertility rates have been falling in most regions of the developing world since 1970, and the latest surveys confirm that fertility has also now begun to fall in sub-Saharan Africa (panel 12). But contrary to the expectations of many, the World Fertility Survey[101] and the Demographic and Health Surveys[102] have revealed that there is still a very high level of unmet demand for family planning in almost all developing countries (fig. 20). At any one time, for example, there are an estimated 120 million women in the developing world who do not want another pregnancy but who have no access to an effective method of contraception.[103] As a result, at least one pregnancy in five in the developing world is unplanned and unwanted.[104]

It is now widely recognized that ris-

ing levels of female education, falling child death rates, and increasing incomes are the main forces which lead people to want fewer children. Family planning services allow people to exercise that choice more easily, and the availability of such services can therefore help to more quickly translate changing circumstances and attitudes into lower fertility rates,[105] so minimizing the time-lag between falling death rates and falling birth rates.

Worlds of difference

Taken together, the improvement of child survival, health, education, and family planning services could have a decisive impact on the PPE problem in the years ahead. To put approximate figures on that impact, reaching all of these goals could make the difference between a world population which stabilizes about a century from now at a level of approximately 10 billion people, and a world population which stabilizes half a century later at a total of around 20 billion.[106] This difference – roughly equivalent to double the entire population of the world in 1993 – may well be sufficient to determine success or failure in managing the transition to a sustainable future.

All of this stands in almost absurd contrast to the smallness of the resources required. The extra amount needed to make family planning generally available by the end of this decade would be approximately $3 billion to $5 billion a year – roughly a doubling of present spending.[107] Today's family planning services account for less than half of 1% of government budgets in the developing world, and less than 1.5% of all aid from governments in the industrialized world.[108] In real terms, international support for family planning services has not increased for approximately 20 years, though there is some encouragement to be drawn from the fact that the United States has now reversed its policies of the 1980s and is once more supporting the efforts of UNFPA, the world's leading international agency for family planning.[109]

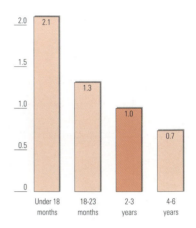

Fig. 18 Space to live

Relative risk of dying before the age of five by interval since the birth of a previous child. Based on a risk factor of 1 when previous child was born 2-3 years earlier.

Source: *John Hobcraft, 'Child spacing and child mortality', Proceedings of the Demographic and Health Surveys World Conference, vol. 2, IRD/Macro International, 1991. Data from 25 countries.*

Fig. 19 Mothers too young

Relative risk of dying before the age of five by age of mother.

Based on a risk factor of 1 when mother is 20-34 years old.

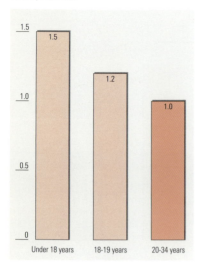

Source: *John Hobcraft, 'Child spacing and child mortality', Proceedings of the Demographic and Health Surveys World Conference, vol. 2, IRD/Macro International, 1991. Data from 18 countries.*

It is too early to say whether governments and the international community will summon the resources and the commitment to reach the family planning goal. But it is not too early to conclude that failure to respond adequately to such an obvious, crucial, and affordable goal will be a clear sign that present political systems and institutions are not equal to the task of managing the great transition.

SYNERGISMS

So far, this chapter has looked at three areas of potential improvement – health and nutrition, basic education, and family planning – from the point of view of their individual impacts on the problems of poverty, population growth and environmental deterioration. But just as there is a destructive synergism among these elements of the PPE spiral, so there is also a constructive synergism between the different elements which contribute to its solution.

The effect of achieving *all* of the basic human goals which have been established would therefore be many times greater than the sum of their individual consequences. And it is this synergism of solutions which offers hope that the achievement of such goals, along with the many other changes that are necessary, will represent a response powerful enough to make a significant difference to the human outcome.

The diagram on page 49 summarizes the most obvious of these synergisms. Many of the relationships it depicts are, in effect, upward spirals of the kind which can multiply several times over the impact of the original improvement. For example:

☐ Family planning is a major contributor to lower under-five mortality rates; lower under-five mortality rates are a major contributor to increased demand for family planning;[110]

☐ Education, particularly of women, means that births are likely to be fewer and better spaced; smaller families mean that children are more likely to become educated (both because their parents can afford the costs of educat-

ing a smaller number of children and because there are fewer siblings and less need for the older ones to look after the younger);[111]

☐ The children of smaller families are generally healthier and better nourished. Better nutritional health means better returns from investments in education. Many hundreds of millions of children are not benefiting from schooling as much as they should because malnutrition affects mental development, or because iodine deficiency means that they are retarded, or because poor nutritional health means poor concentration, or because frequent illness means that a significant percentage of school days are missed altogether;

☐ Similarly, better education helps to ensure better health. Not only are educated families likely to absorb more health knowledge and be more aware of the importance of hygiene and preventive health measures, they have also been shown to be much more likely to demand and to use private or public health services.[112]

Taken together, these mutually reinforcing relationships lead to smaller families and healthier, better-educated children. This in turn means that those children are better able to respond to new opportunities and to earn a living for themselves and their own families, so that their own children are also likely to enjoy better nutrition, health, and education. This virtuous cycle has demonstrated its power in such diverse societies as China, the Republic of Korea, Sri Lanka, and Taiwan. And as figure 21 shows, the countries and regions which gave priority to these investments in people in the 1950s and 1960s have succeeded in controlling population growth, and will eventually stabilize their populations at much lower levels than would otherwise have been the case.

These and the many other mutually reinforcing effects of reaching basic human goals hold out the hope that an upward spiral can be substituted for the downward. Along with the creation of wider employment opportunities, it is investments in reaching basic

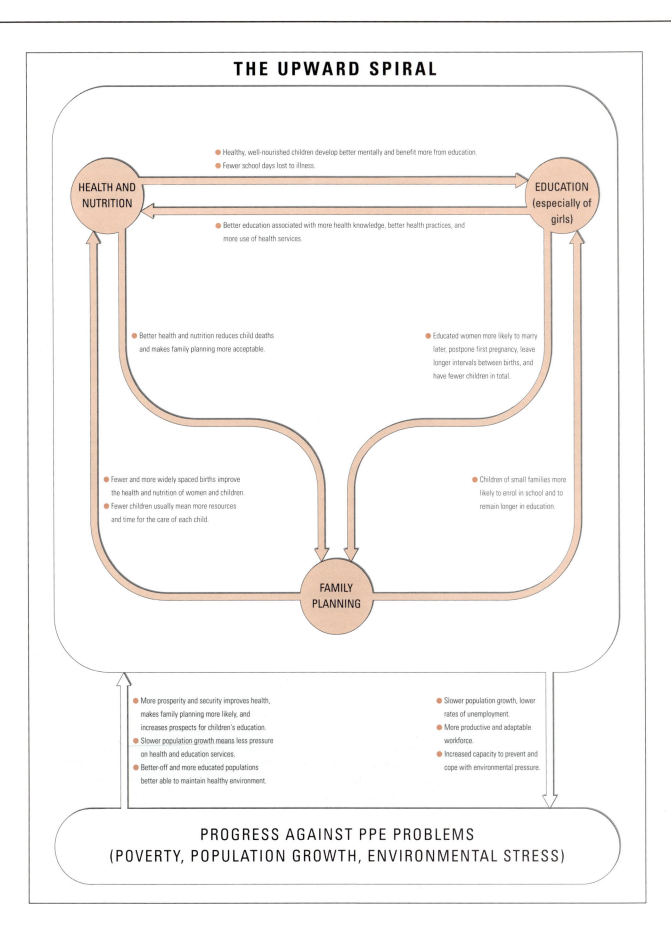

THE UPWARD SPIRAL

HEALTH AND NUTRITION

● Healthy, well-nourished children develop better mentally and benefit more from education.
● Fewer school days lost to illness.

EDUCATION (especially of girls)

● Better education associated with more health knowledge, better health practices, and more use of health services.

● Better health and nutrition reduces child deaths and makes family planning more acceptable.

● Educated women more likely to marry later, postpone first pregnancy, leave longer intervals between births, and have fewer children in total.

● Fewer and more widely spaced births improve the health and nutrition of women and children.
● Fewer children usually mean more resources and time for the care of each child.

● Children of small families more likely to enrol in school and to remain longer in education.

FAMILY PLANNING

● More prosperity and security improves health, makes family planning more likely, and increases prospects for children's education.
● Slower population growth means less pressure on health and education services.
● Better-off and more educated populations better able to maintain healthy environment.

● Slower population growth, lower rates of unemployment.
● More productive and adaptable workforce.
● Increased capacity to prevent and cope with environmental pressure.

PROGRESS AGAINST PPE PROBLEMS
(POVERTY, POPULATION GROWTH, ENVIRONMENTAL STRESS)

Fig. 20 Unmet demand

Married women who do not want to become pregnant – percentages using and not using contraception.

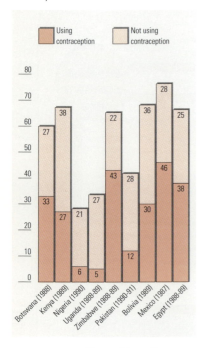

Using contraception   Not using contraception

The unmet demand for contraception includes demand for both spacing births and limiting family size.

Source: *Demographic and Health Surveys cited in 'The reproductive revolution; new survey findings',* Population Reports, *series M, no. 11, December 1992.*

human goals that offer the best chance of reversing the PPE spiral.

Putting the basic benefits of progress at the disposal of all communities is therefore the best that the 1990s can do both for today's children – and for tomorrow's world.

AFRICA

It is impossible to conclude this review of the present potential and present threats without special mention of the problems of sub-Saharan Africa.

Examined through all three of the lenses used in this report – poverty, population, and environment – the position of Africa is cause for the greatest concern.

Economically, Africa has begun sliding backwards into poverty. In the 1980s, its per capita GNP declined by almost 2% a year, leaving the average citizen significantly poorer by the end of the decade. In total, about 220 million Africans – almost half of the population south of the Sahara – now live in absolute poverty, unable to meet their most basic needs.[113]

As a result, malnutrition has increased in some African nations, even as it has been declining in most other regions of the world. In some regions of Zambia, according to a 1993 report by the voluntary agency OXFAM, the proportion of children who are malnourished has risen from 5% to 25% in the last decade.[114] Health services have also declined in many of the hardest-hit nations, though extraordinary efforts have been made to lift immunization coverage from less than 20% to approximately 60% since 1985 (with 11 African countries surpassing the 70% mark for vaccination against measles). In education, also, the 1980s can only be described as a lost decade as expenditure per student declined by about one third, primary school enrolment fell from 79% to 67%,[115] and an estimated one third of all college graduates left the continent.[116] As if these problems were not enough, many millions of African families today are being devastated and many children orphaned by AIDS (panel 13).

As well as the suffering caused by conflict and worsening poverty, Africa has also been the scene for the most terrible enactment of the environmental processes described in part 2 of this report: soil erosion now affects more than three quarters of all cultivable land; tropical forests are being destroyed at a rate of 5 million hectares a year; and 80% to 90% of the sub-Sahelian zone, the Sudan, and the northern parts of Ethiopia and Kenya are degraded by erosion and the loss of trees and scrub, leading to further erosion and further falls in yields.[117] In total, at least 30 million people are so severely affected by these processes as to be under almost constant threat of drought and starvation. "*No other region*," said the Brundtland Commission, "*more tragically suffers the vicious cycle of poverty leading to environmental degradation, which leads in turn to even greater poverty.*"[118]

Current forecasts of population growth are sobering, even for the emptiest continent. The total population of Africa south of the Sahara is projected to rise from 0.6 billion today to 1.6 billion by the year 2030.[119] Nearly 30 African nations, including Ethiopia, Kenya, Nigeria, Uganda, Tanzania and Zaire, are set to double their present populations in less than 25 years.[120]

Debt defeats development

The causes and potential solutions of Africa's problems have been analysed in detail in several other United Nations publications,[121] and it will be sufficient here to make brief mention of the main points.

First, a weak trading position, caused by dependence on a small range of primary commodities, by internal mismanagement, and by trade and tariff barriers which hinder diversification,[122] has meant that Africa's share of world trade has declined from almost 4% to 1% in the 1980s. Falling prices for the continent's main export commodities, in particular, have meant losses of approximately $12 billion a year. In Côte d'Ivoire, for example, exports of coffee rose by 26% in volume but fell by 21% in value between 1988 and 1990.[123]

Second, the combination of internal conflicts and cold war fostering of dictatorships has led to the militarization of the continent. The result has been devastating. A vast proportion of Africa's resources, and of external aid, has been diverted to military purposes. In addition, military conflicts, fuelled by an excess of weaponry, have damaged the future prospects and present livelihoods of many tens of millions of African families. At a minimum, 7.5 million to 10 million households in sub-Saharan Africa have had their livelihoods wiped out by wars and conflicts in recent years[124] and many millions more have become refugees.

Third, Africa has also been devastated by debt. As figure 22 shows, sub-Saharan Africa bears a far heavier debt burden than any other region of the developing world. Each year, repayments of capital and interest totalling over $30 billion fall due. Only about one third of this is actually paid. The rest is simply added to the total owed, a total which almost trebled in the 1980s.[125] But even this annual repayment of more than $10 billion is a crippling burden, amounting to four times as much as Africa spends on its health services and far more than is spent on the health and education of its children.[126]

To put this problem of debt into the overall context of this year's *State of the World's Children* report, the total cost of meeting the basic human goals in Africa – for health, nutrition, education, and family planning – would be approximately $9 billion a year; this is significantly less than Africa is currently finding for the sake of paying off one third of the interest due on a colossal burden of debt most of which, as every expert agrees, can never be repaid.

In addition to the mistakes of its own leaders, Africa has therefore been further exploited by the outside world in its hour of greatest need. The suffering and loss has been incalculable, a financial holocaust from which Africa cannot recover without an international effort on a scale that has not yet been contemplated.

Solutions

The actions required to halt and reverse the decline of sub-Saharan Africa are as well known as the problems themselves.

First, as UNICEF and many non-governmental organizations have repeatedly argued,[127] Africa's debts must be drastically written down. Debt relief should include moneys owed to the governments of industrialized countries (three quarters of Africa's total debt) and to the World Bank and the International Monetary Fund. In particular, debt relief schemes should result in major reductions in the actual amount that Africa pays out on its debts each year (so far, most of the limited debt cancellation has applied to debts which were not being serviced anyway). Wherever possible, debt relief should also be linked to reductions in military spending, and to increases in expenditures designed to achieve basic human goals in health, nutrition, education, and family planning.

Second, Africa's trading position must be allowed to become stronger, through agreement on reasonable and stable prices for commodities, through the lowering of trade barriers to Africa's processed and manufactured goods, through the creation of an economic diversification fund, and through increased aid and investment.

Third, military spending must decline more steeply. This is primarily the responsibility of African governments – governments that will be judged harshly by the rest of the world if they continue to divert to military purposes the resources that should be invested in job creation, environmental protection, family planning, and the health, education, and nutrition of Africa's children. But it is also the responsibility of governments in the industrialized nations who support the export of arms to Africa. As the Secretary-General of the United Nations has said: "*Those who provide arms could be considered as partners to the crime. The flow of arms to the developing world must be stopped.*"[128]

Fourth, African governments must

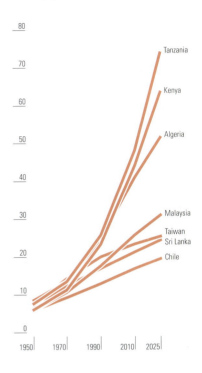

Fig. 21 Population paths

Actual and projected populations (in millions) for seven countries that had approximately the same population in 1950.

Tanzania
Kenya
Algeria
Malaysia
Taiwan
Sri Lanka
Chile

80
70
60
50
40
30
20
10
0

1950 1970 1990 2010 2025

Sources: *United Nations,* World population prospects: the 1992 revision, *1993. Data for Taiwan from World Bank, 1993.*

Fig. 22 Debt burden

Total debt as percentage of GNP, 1991.

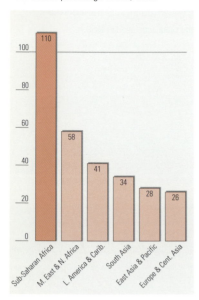

Source: *World Bank*, World debt tables 1992-93, vol. 1, 1992.

make good the commitments they have made to invest a greater proportion of their revenues in human resources, and to achieve the basic human goals that have been established in the fields of health, nutrition, education, and family planning.[129] In Dakar in 1992, and again in Cairo in 1993, Africa's political leaders have declared their intention of reaching these goals by the end of this decade. Those commitments should now be met by corresponding commitments of extra resources, for these specific purposes, from the industrialized nations.

Fifth, the international community should assist Africa in its struggle towards democracy not only through cooperation to strengthen Africa's economic position, and support for African governments' commitments to the achievement of basic human goals, but also through direct assistance to those policies and institutions which deepen democracy's foundations. This issue, too, has been recently addressed by the Secretary-General of the United Nations:

"Time and again, all across Africa, hopeful steps towards development have stopped because of instability. This cycle can be broken only through the growth of democratic practices...

"Development aid must include support for the creation and strengthening of institutions of democracy. Democracy should be understood as the move towards better, more participatory government, perceived as such by the governed. Unless democracy takes root, violence, coups d'état, wars and general instability will recur, with an inevitable effect on socio-economic development."[130]

Signs of change

The situation in Africa can be turned round. Fundamental changes, emerging from this last disastrous decade, have created a different and far more hopeful framework for African development. In the last five years, many African countries have undertaken fundamental reforms. There is an almost continent-wide movement towards democracy, however frustrating and

difficult that journey may be. Apartheid is coming to an end. Economies have been liberalized. The climate for investment is improving. The cold war no longer nurtures dictatorships. Several long-running wars have been ended or scaled down. Military spending, in at least some countries, is showing signs of decline.[131] And most of Africa's political leaders committed themselves and their governments to the meeting of basic human goals.[132]

There are also early signs of a possible change in attitudes in the industrialized nations. United States Secretary of State Warren Christopher has said that cold war interests will now be replaced, at the heart of America's relationship with Africa, by *"an enduring commitment to democracy and human rights"*.[133] Similarly, President Clinton has acknowledged that *"A revolution is under way in Africa... Africans are struggling to achieve political and economic freedoms... We have a strong interest in helping them translate those freedoms into a better life for themselves and their children."*[134] European leaders have made similar statements and several industrialized nations have moved to link the continuation of aid programmes to progress towards democracy and reductions in military spending.

These are all signs of hope. But it must be said that so far there has been little sign of action by the industrialized countries, and that threatening cuts in aid, however justifiable and necessary it might be, is not an adequate response to the crisis of sub-Saharan Africa. And if, after many decades of offering moral, material, and military support to often blatantly corrupt and repressive dictatorships, the industrialized nations now wish to foster 'good governance' in Africa, then they must also act to strengthen Africa's economic position by writing off many of the subcontinent's debts, by agreeing fair and stable prices for its raw materials, by reducing tariffs on Africa's manufactured exports,[135] and by increasing the amount of aid available for investing in Africa's people and meeting basic human goals.

RETHINK

As the great problems discussed in this report come slowly into clearer focus, there is an increasing recognition that managing the transition to a sustainable future should become the new central organizing principle of the post-cold war era. There is also a growing awareness that coming to grips with the great crises of poverty, population growth, and environmental deterioration in the poorest regions of the globe is an essential part of that transition.

The broad outlines of the response that is required are being embraced by academic experts, by international agencies, by non-governmental organizations, by many in the media, and by some political parties and leaders.

As part of that response, the cause of meeting the basic human needs of the poorest quarter of humanity must be taken up with a new determination both for its own sake and as a means of pre-empting PPE problems which will increasingly affect not only the poorest communities but the prospects for democracy, economic advance, and political stability within and between nations.

At the same time, the gains that have been made in many parts of the developing world must be protected from environmental threats, and those large areas of the world which are achieving economic growth must be enabled to fulfil their legitimate material aspirations without exceeding the earth's capacity to provide, absorb, and regenerate.

To achieve this, it will be necessary for the industrialized nations to move on three broad fronts:

☐ To create an 'enabling' rather than 'disabling' international economic environment within which the developing world can achieve economic growth. In practice, this would mean agreements on fair and stable commodity prices, agreements on more open access to markets for the manufactured exports from poor countries, agreements to write down a significant proportion of debt in selected regions and cases, and a renewal of aid and investment with the emphasis on investing in the health and education and employment of the poorest;

☐ To undertake intensive research efforts, in cooperation with scientists and technicians from developing countries, in order to develop and deploy the kind of technologies which will raise living standards and fulfil legitimate aspirations without endangering the biosphere;

☐ To rethink their own definition of progress in order to improve the quality of life while reducing impact on the biosphere. One test of any new definition of progress will be whether or not its pattern of consumption and pollution would be environmentally sustainable even if similar levels of progress were attained by all nations.

Democracy's challenge

Throughout the world, voices are growing in support of a new effort to focus national and international action on these new challenges in the post-cold war period. Frequently, those voices refer back to a previous occasion, almost half a century ago, when crisis and chaos threatened the industrialized world in the aftermath of the Second World War. They refer, specifically, to the day in June of 1947 when General George Marshall outlined a plan which stands to this day as one of the most outstanding examples in human history of the generosity of spirit, the far-sighted practicality, and the willingness to dream and act on the grand scale that are the fundamental prerequisites of successfully managing the transition which must now be made.

As its architect foresaw, the Marshall Plan succeeded in helping to build democracy and prosperity not only in Europe but in the wider world, with the United States itself being one of the principal long-term beneficiaries. "*The Marshall Plan*," writes the Vice-President of the United States, "*took the broadest possible view of Europe's problems and developed strategies to serve human needs and promote sustained economic progress; we must now do the*

The industrialized countries must rethink their own definition of progress in order to improve the quality of life while reducing their impact on the biosphere.

The most basic advantages of progress have not yet been made available to the poorest fifth of human society.

same on a global scale."[136]

But there is as yet little sign that the industrialized world is prepared to act with an equivalent boldness and vision in the face of present challenges.

Ultimately, the barrier to such action, the barrier that separates humanity from a sustainable future, is not financial or technical or environmental. It is at heart a political barrier. There is very little doubt that the world has the resources and the ingenuity to make the transition to a world in which the basic needs of every man, woman and child are met and in which the human adventure – with all its potential for progress, growth, change, excitement, discovery – can continue. What is in question is the capacity of our institutions and political systems to respond to these entirely new challenges. For as most of the world makes progress away from totalitarianism, it is becoming increasingly clear that democracy itself is not working adequately as a means of resolving longer-term problems. The focus of political life in the established democracies appears essentially narrow and short term. As a result, political vision often appears to be circumscribed by opinion polls, and to extend only as far as the next election, whereas the widely acknowledged problems which threaten our own and our children's futures require vision and action on a different scale in both place and time. This problem of dysfunction between political institutions and the problems that they are required to resolve is not one that was faced or even contemplated by those who originally framed the articles of democracy; but it is one which will have to be grappled with by those who must now use them to manage a global transition of an unprecedented complexity.

This is a contradiction which must be resolved, as such intractable problems have been in the past, by a change in the prevailing climate of ideas, in the underlying ethic that ultimately shapes public perceptions and political priorities. It is this process – led more often by people than by governments – that has gradually dislodged such entrenched concepts and institutions as slavery and colonialism, apartheid and racism. And it is this process that, in more recent times, has begun to bring about profound changes in our attitudes towards the natural environment or towards the rights and status of women.

Looked at from the perspective of several decades rather than from the platform of months or years, the possibility of such change, and its immense power in the world of practical events, becomes much more obvious. Up until this century, for example, almost all societies were organized in the interests of a relatively narrow élite who enjoyed an almost exclusive monopoly of rights and privileges, and of the benefits of progress. For the most part, this state of affairs went unquestioned, being almost universally regarded as normal, as a reflection of some preordained order: aristocrat over peasant, employer over worker, white race over black, European over African and Asian, male over female. The practical consequences of that prevailing ethic, with all its entrenched injustices and inequalities, are still very much with us. But it is equally undeniable that a profound change in the underlying ethic, in what is considered acceptable, has occurred. Few today would not accept, at least in principle, that all people should have the same rights and opportunities, or that the basic benefits of progress should be available to all.

This change in ethos has begun to change the world of events and institutions, and is slowly becoming the heart of humanity's struggle for progress.

But in one area, above all, the application of this changing ethic lags badly behind. The most basic rights, the most basic opportunities, and the most basic advantages of progress have not yet been made available to the more than 1 billion people who make up the poorest fifth of human society. That is the most glaring deficiency in human progress and human civilization as we near the end of the 20th century.

Yet it is possible today, amid all the conflicts and atrocities, to see the beginnings of the kind of change in ethos which may one day make good this deficiency. Through the dust and debris of the immediate shocks, disasters, and set-backs of the present day, it is not always easy to see that underlying change in the ethical landscape. Yet looked at over a period of several decades, such a change becomes more obvious. Fifty years ago this year, 1.5 million people starved to death in a famine in Bengal while the outside world knew little and did less.[137]

Today, when famine strikes, a worldwide public knows more and cares more, and is unprepared to tolerate mass deaths and suffering on its television screens. The result is that governments are obliged to take action. And however belated and inadequate such action may be, it nonetheless reflects the beginnings of an important shift in the underlying ethic, in what is considered acceptable in the world and what is not.

Similarly, the international intervention in Somalia, for all its difficulties and set-backs, nonetheless represents a first declaration that the international community will not stand by and do nothing while the people – and the children – of a failed state succumb to mass suffering and starvation.

But so far, this new ethic has been limited to sudden and well-publicized set-backs and disasters; it has not yet been extended to the 'silent emergencies' of mass malnutrition, disease, and illiteracy which inflict both immediate suffering and lifelong consequences on even larger numbers of people.

The challenge of the 1990s is to deepen and broaden the new ethic that is beginning to emerge, in order to also render unacceptable large-scale suffering from these more ordinary, everyday, less spectacular causes. When little could be done about the worst aspects of poverty, it was perhaps forgivable that they should attract so little attention and be accorded so little priority. But almost without the world noticing, advances in knowledge and outreach capacity have made it possible to bring to an end the worst aspects of poverty that crush human lives and human potential and give such impetus to the problems of poverty, population growth, and environmental deterioration. If this all-important change in the underlying ethos is to be completed, and if the transition to a sustainable future is to be made, then it is essential that people and their organizations, in all countries, should also become intolerant of the unnecessary suffering involved in the larger-scale but lesser-known tragedies of mass malnutrition and disease, illiteracy and disability.

Only such a change can give the task of meeting minimum human needs the sustained priority it deserves. Only such a change can ensure that political leaderships keep faith with the promises that have been made. And only such a change will ensure that what can now be done will now be done – and that the evils of mass malnutrition, disease, and illiteracy are brought to an end in our times. □

The year 2000: what can be achieved?

The following is the full list of year 2000 goals which the world's political leaders agreed upon – as being technically and financially feasible – at the World Summit for Children on 30 September 1990.

Overall goals 1990-2000

☐ A one-third reduction in under-five death rates (or a reduction to 70 per 1,000 live births – whichever is lower).

☐ A halving of maternal mortality rates.

☐ A halving of severe and moderate malnutrition among the world's under-fives.

☐ Safe water and sanitation for all families.

☐ Basic education for all children and completion of primary education by at least 80%.

☐ A halving of the adult illiteracy rate and the achievement of equal educational opportunity for males and females.

☐ Protection for the many millions of children in especially difficult circumstances and the acceptance and observance, in all countries, of the recently adopted Convention on the Rights of the Child. In particular, the 1990s should see rapidly growing acceptance of the idea of special protection for children in time of war.

Protection for girls and women

☐ Family planning education and services to be made available to all couples to empower them to prevent unwanted pregnancies and births which are 'too many and too close' and to women who are 'too young or too old'. Such services should be adapted to each country's cultural, religious, and social traditions.

☐ All women to have access to prenatal care, a trained attendant during childbirth and referral facilities for high-risk pregnancies and obstetric emergencies.

☐ Universal recognition of the special health and nutritional needs of females during early childhood, adolescence, pregnancy, and lactation.

Nutrition

☐ A reduction in the incidence of low birth weight (under 2.5 kg) to less than 10%.

☐ A one-third reduction in iron deficiency anaemia among women.

☐ Virtual elimination of vitamin A deficiency and iodine deficiency disorders.

☐ All families to know the importance of supporting women in the task of exclusive breastfeeding for the first four to six months of a child's life.

☐ Growth monitoring and promotion to be institutionalized in all countries.

☐ Dissemination of knowledge to enable all families to ensure household food security.

Child health

☐ The eradication of polio.

☐ The elimination of neonatal tetanus (by 1995).

☐ A 90% reduction in measles cases and a 95% reduction in measles deaths, compared to pre-immunization levels.

☐ Achievement and maintenance of at least 90% immunization coverage of one-year-old children and universal tetanus immunization for women in the child-bearing years.

☐ A halving of child deaths caused by diarrhoea and a 25% reduction in the incidence of diarrhoeal diseases.

☐ A one-third reduction in child deaths caused by acute respiratory infections.

☐ The elimination of guinea worm disease.

Education

☐ In addition to the expansion of primary school education and its equivalents, today's essential knowledge and life skills could be put at the disposal of all families by mobilizing today's vastly increased communications capacity.

MID-DECADE GOALS

In order to maintain a sense of urgency, most of the developing world's governments have also agreed to try to reach a limited number of goals by the middle of the decade. The following are considered achievable by the end of 1995:

☐ Elimination of neonatal tetanus

☐ Reduction of measles morbidity by 90%

☐ Reduction of measles mortality by 95%

☐ Achievement of 80% ORT use for diarrhoeal disease

☐ Eradication of polio (certain countries)

☐ Elimination of iodine deficiency disorders

☐ Success of the 'baby-friendly hospital initiative'

☐ Elimination of vitamin A deficiency

☐ Elimination of guinea worm

☐ Achievement of 80% immunization in all countries

REFERENCES

1   United Nations Children's Fund, *The State of the World's Children 1993*, UNICEF, New York, p. 5
2   *Dialogue on Diarrhoea*, No. 52, March-May 1993, Appropriate Health Resources and Technologies Action Group (AHRTAG), London
3   World Health Organization, Programme for Control of Diarrhoeal Diseases, *Interim Programme Report 1992*, WHO/CDD/93.40, WHO, Geneva, 1992
4   Figures supplied by World Health Organization, Geneva, August 1993
5   Ibid.
6   Ibid.
7   World Health Organization, *The International Drinking Water Supply and Sanitation Decade: End of Decade Review*, WHO/CWS/92.12, WHO, Geneva, 1992
    World Health Organization and United Nations Children's Fund, *Water Supply and Sanitation Sector Monitoring Report 1993*, WHO/UNICEF Joint Monitoring Programme, Geneva and New York, 1993
8   Ibid.
9   World Health Organization, *Reproductive Health: A Key to a Brighter Future. Biennial Report 1990-1991*, WHO, Geneva, 1992
10 United Nations Children's Fund, *The Progress of Nations 1993*, UNICEF, New York, 1993, p. 34
11 World Health Organization, Press Release No.45, WHO, Geneva, 22 June 1992
12 Mahalanabis, Dilip, 'The Pioneering Years', *Dialogue on Diarrhoea*, No. 52, March-May 1993, p. 5
13 United Nations Administrative Committee on Coordination, Subcommittee on Nutrition, *Second Report on the World Nutrition Situation*, United Nations, New York, 1992, p. 39
14 United Nations Children's Fund, Nutrition Cluster, 'A UNICEF Strategy for the Control of Iodine Deficiency Disorders', UNICEF, New York, September 1993
15 Levine, Ruth E., and others, 'Breast-feeding Saves Lives: An Estimate of Breastfeeding-related Infant Survival', Center to Prevent Childhood Malnutrition, Maryland, USA, 31 May 1990
16 World Bank, *World Development Report 1993*, World Bank, Washington, D.C., 1993, p. 93
    United Nations Children's Fund, 'Strategies and Resources: Operational Strategy Framework for Dracunculiasis Eradication', UNICEF, New York, July 1992, appendix G-3
17 World Health Organization, *Our Planet, Our Health*, WHO, Geneva, 1992, p. 122
18 Yambi, Olivia, and Mlolwa, Raphael, *Improving Nutrition in Tanzania in the 1980s: The Iringa Experience*, UNICEF, International Child Development Centre, Florence, Innocenti Occasional Papers No. 25, March 1992
19 World Health Organization, *Maternal Mortality: A Global Factbook*, WHO, Geneva, 1991
    United Nations Children's Fund, *The Progress of Nations 1993*, op. cit., p.39
20 United Nations Children's Fund, 'World Declaration on the Survival, Protection and Development of Children' and 'Plan of Action for Implementing the World Declaration on the Survival, Protection and Development of Children in the 1990s', UNICEF, New York, 1990
21 Data supplied by World Health Organization, August 1993
22 Ibid.
23 World Health Organization, Expanded Programme on Immunization, *Programme Report 1992*, WHO/EPI/GEN/93.1, WHO, Geneva, January 1993, p. 6
24 Ibid.
25 Ibid., p. 30
26 United Nations Children's Fund, Nutrition Cluster, op. cit.
27 United Nations Children's Fund and World Health Organization, 'Progress Report to the Joint Committee on Health Policy', JCHP29/93.1, UNICEF-WHO Joint Committee on Health Policy, 29th session, Geneva, February 1993
28 World Health Organization and United Nations Children's Fund, 'Protecting, Promoting and Supporting Breast-feeding: The Special Role of Maternity Services', joint WHO/UNICEF statement, WHO, Geneva, 1989
29 Gonzales, Ricardo B., 'A Large-scale Rooming-in Program in a Developing Country: The Dr. Jose Fabella Memorial Hospital Experience', Manila, December 1988. Available from UNICEF, Nutrition Cluster, New York
30 *IRC Newsletter*, No. 215, March 1993, International Water and Sanitation Centre, The Hague, p. 2
    Countdown, Vol. 1, No. 3, October 1992, UNICEF, Programme Division, New York, p. 2
31 World Bank, *World Development Report 1993*, op. cit., p. 114
32 United Nations Children's Fund and World Health Organization, 'The World Summit for Children: An Overview of Follow-up Action in Health, 1993-1995', JCHP29/93.3, UNICEF-WHO Joint Committee on Health Policy, 29th session, Geneva, February 1993
33 'Water with Sugar and Salt', *The Lancet*, 5 August 1978, p. 300
34 World Health Organization, Expanded Programme on Immunization, op. cit., p. 7
35 World Health Organization, *Maternal Mortality: A Global Factbook*, op. cit.
36 'The Reproductive Revolution: New Survey Findings', *Population Reports*, Series M, No. 11, Population Information Program, Johns Hopkins University, Baltimore, December 1992
37 United Nations Children's Fund, *The Progress of Nations 1993*, op. cit.
38 United Nations Development Programme, *Human Development Report 1993*, UNDP, New York, 1993
39 United Nations Development Programme, *Human Development Report 1992*, UNDP, New York, 1992, p. 45
40 Figures supplied by Programme Funding Office, UNICEF, New York
41 United Nations Children's Fund, *The Progress of Nations 1993*, op. cit., p. 18
42 United Nations Development Programme, *Human Development Report 1993*, op. cit., overview and chapter 2
43 United Nations Children's Fund, Division of Information, survey of public opinion polls conducted in Canada, the European Community and the United States, UNICEF, New York
44 United Nations Development Programme, *Human Development Report 1993*, op. cit., p. 7
    United States aid: Nowels, Larry Q., 'Foreign Aid: Clinton Administration Budget and Policy Initiative'; Congressional Research Service, Washington, D.C., 7 October 1993
45 Deger, Saadet, *The Economics of Disarmament: Prospects, Problems and Policies for the Disarmament Dividend*, UNICEF, International Child Development Centre, Florence, Innocenti Occasional Papers, Economic Policy Series, No. 30, August 1992, p. 10

46 United Nations, *Long-range World Population Projections: Two Centuries of Population Growth 1950-2150*, United Nations, New York, 1992

47 Durning, Alan, 'Asking How Much is Enough', in *The State of the World 1991*, Worldwatch Institute, Norton/Worldwatch books, Washington, D.C., 1991

48 Ross, John A., and others, *Family Planning and Child Survival Programs as Assessed in 1991*, Population Council, New York, 1992

49 LeVine, Robert A., and others, 'Women's Schooling and Child Care in the Demographic Transition: A Mexican Case Study', *Population and Development Review*, Vol. 17, No. 3, September 1991

50 Clay, Daniel C., and Vander Haar, Jane E., 'Patterns of Intergenerational Support and Childbearing in the Third World', *Population Studies*, Vol. 47, 1993

51 Ibid.

52 United Nations, Department of International Economic and Social Affairs, 'Family Building by Fate or Design: A Study of Relationships between Child Survival and Fertility', ST/ESA/SER.R/74, United Nations, New York, 1987

53 Havanon, Napaporn, Knodel, John, and Sittitrai, Werasit, 'The Impact of Family Size on Wealth Accumulation in Rural Thailand', *Population Studies*, Vol. 46, 1992

54 Leonard, Jeffrey, ed., *Environment and the Poor: Development Strategies for a Common Agenda*, Overseas Development Council, Washington, D.C., 1989 World Commission on Environment and Development (Brundtland Commission), *Our Common Future*, Oxford University Press, 1987

55 United Nations Development Programme, *Human Development Report 1992*, op. cit.

56 Brogan, Hugh, *The Pelican History of the United States*, Penguin Books/Viking, 1987

57 Kennedy, Paul, *Preparing for the Twenty-first Century*, Random House, New York, 1993

58 Leonard, Jeffrey, ed., op. cit., p. 25

59 OXFAM, *Africa: Action for Recovery*, Oxford, April 1993, p. 32

60 World Food Council, 'Sustainable Food Security: Action for Environmental Management of Agriculture', WFC/1988/5/Add.1, WFC, Rome, 1988, p. 5

61 Food and Agriculture Organization of the United Nations, *The State of Food and Agriculture*, FAO, Rome, 1991 and 1992 reports

62 Overseas Development Council, 'Growth from Below: A People-oriented Development Strategy', Development Paper No. 16, ODC, Washington, D.C., December 1973

63 World Commission on Environment and Development (Brundtland Commission), op. cit., p. 29

64 De Boer, John, 'Sustainable Approaches to Hillside Agricultural Development', in Leonard, Jeffrey, ed., op. cit.

65 Statement by His Excellency Dr. Kofi N. Awoonor, Ambassador of Ghana to the United Nations, address to the Group of 77, United Nations, 1 October 1991

66 Secretary-General of the United Nations, *An Agenda for Peace*, A/47/277-S/24111, United Nations, New York, 1992

67 Kennedy, Paul, op. cit., p. 11

68 United Nations Population Fund, *The State of World Population 1993*, UNFPA, New York, 1993

69 Ibid.

70 Ehrlich, Paul R., and Ehrlich, Anne H., *The Population Explosion*, Simon and Schuster, New York, 1990, p. 134

71 Agenda 21, report of the United Nations Conference on Environment and Development to the General Assembly of the United Nations, sales number 93.1.11, United Nations, New York, 1993 World Commission on Environment and Development (Brundtland Commission), op. cit.

72 World Commission on Environment and Development (Brundtland Commission), op. cit.

73 'A Green Wall', *The Economist*, 11 April 1992

74 Meadows, D.H., Meadows, D.L., and Rendels, J., *Beyond the Limits: Global Collapse or a Sustainable Future*, Earthscan Publications, London, 1992, pp. 210-211

75 For a discussion of some of the necessary environmental investments in marginal agricultural areas, see Leonard, Jeffrey, ed., op. cit., pp. 29-31 and 38-39

76 Eliasson, Jan, 'Enlarging the United Nations' Humanitarian Mandate', DPI/1320, United Nations, New York, December 1992

77 Kennedy, Paul, op. cit., pp. 14-15

78 Rotfeld, Adam Daniel, 'The Fundamental Changes and the New Security Agenda', in *World Armaments and Disarmament*, yearbook of the Stockholm International Peace Research Institute, Stockholm, 1992

79 Gore, Al, *Earth in the Balance*, Plume Books, New York, 1993, p. 31

80 Goldmark, Peter C., Jr., President, Rockefeller Foundation, speech to the Overseas Development Council, Washington, D.C., June 1991

81 Gore, Al, op. cit., pp. 297-307

82 World Bank, *World Development Report 1993*, op. cit. This year's report, subtitled 'Investing in Health', examines the interplay between human health, health policy and economic development

83 Ibid., p. 2

84 Ross, John A., and others, op. cit. Rashad, Hoda, El Bahy, Mohamed, and Attia, Shadia, 'Linking Fertility Change to Community-level Changes in Mortality: The Egyptian Case', study carried out for UNICEF by the Population Council, West Asia and North Africa Office, 1992

85 Akhter, Halida H., and Saifuddin, Ahmed, 'Determinants of Contraceptive Continuation in Rural Bangladesh', *Journal of Biosocial Science*, Vol. 24, No. 2, 1992

86 Ross, John A., and others, op. cit.

87 United Nations, Department of International Economic and Social Affairs, 'Family Building by Fate or Design: A Study of Relationships between Child Survival and Fertility', op. cit.

88 Ibid.

89 United Nations Children's Fund, *The Progress of Nations 1993*, op. cit., p. 35

90 Carnoy, Martin, *The Case for Investing in Basic Education*, UNICEF, New York, 1992, p. 26

91 United Nations Development Programme, *Human Development Report 1992*, op. cit., box 4.6, p. 69

92 World Bank, *World Development Report 1992*, World Bank, 1992

93 LeVine, Robert A., and others, 'Women's Schooling and Child Care in the Demographic Transition: A Mexican Case Study', *Population and Development Review*, Vol. 17, No. 3, September 1991

Pillai, Vijayan K., 'Men and Family Planning in Zambia', *Journal of Biosocial Science*, Vol. 25, January 1993

94 Catley-Carlson, Margaret, President, Population Council, 'Explosions, Eclipses and Escapes: Charting a Course on Global Population Issues', 1993 Paul Hoffman Lecture for United Nations Development Programme, New York, 7 June 1993

95 World Bank, *World Development Report 1992*, op. cit., p. 29

96 Catley-Carlson, Margaret, op. cit.

97 Data from United Nations Educational, Scientific and Cultural Organization published in UNICEF, *The Progress of Nations 1993*, op. cit., p. 27

98 Ibid., p. 28

99 Anderson, Mary B., *Education for All: What are we Waiting For?*, UNICEF, New York, 1992
See also Lovell, Catherine H., *Breaking the Cycle of Poverty: The BRAC Strategy*, Kumarian Press, Dhaka, 1992

100 Rowley, John, and Mahler, Halfdan, 'Family Planning Can Contribute to Health for All', in Rohde, Jon, Chatterjee, Meera, and Morley, David, eds., *Reaching Health for All*, Oxford University Press, 1993, p. 474

101 The World Fertility Survey, conducted between 1972 and 1984, was the first worldwide programme to collect comparable national survey statistics on fertility and family planning. For further information see Cleland, John, and others, eds., *The World Fertility Survey: An Assessment*, Oxford University Press, 1987

102 The Demographic and Health Surveys, started in 1985, have continued the work of the World Fertility Survey. Between 1985 and 1992 more than a quarter of a million women were interviewed for the surveys in 36 nations, from questionnaires averaging about 250 questions. For further information see the *DHS Comparative Studies* series, Institute for Resource Development/Macro International, Columbia, Maryland

103 'The Reproductive Revolution: New Survey Findings', op. cit.

104 Westoff, Charles F., 'Reproductive Preferences: A Comparative View', *DHS Comparative Studies*, No. 3, 1991

105 Koenig, Michael A., and others, 'Contraceptive Use in Matlab, Bangladesh 1990: Levels, Trends and Explanations', *Studies in Family Planning*, Vol. 23, No. 6, November-December 1992

106 United Nations, *Long-range World Population Projections: Two Centuries of Population Growth 1950-2150*, op. cit.

107 'The Reproductive Revolution: New Survey Findings', op. cit.

108 United Nations Population Fund, *Global Population Assistance Report 1982-1990*, UNFPA, New York, 1992

109 Rowen, Hobart, '$100 Million More for Family Planning', *The Washington Post*, 24 June 1993

110 Potts, Malcolm, and Thapa, Shyam, *Child Survival: The Role of Family Planning*, Family Health International, North Carolina, September 1991
See also 'Risk Factors: Whether the Pregnancy is Wanted and Mother's Age', *Safe Motherhood*, No. 7, WHO, Division of Family Health, November 1991-February 1992

111 Knodel, John, *Fertility Decline and Children's Education in Thailand: Some Macro and Micro Effects*, Working Paper No. 40, Population Council, New York, 1992

112 World Bank, *World Development Report 1993*, op. cit.

113 World Bank, *World Development Report 1992*, op. cit.

114 OXFAM, op. cit.

115 United Nations Development Programme, *Human Development Report 1992*, op. cit., box 3.1, p. 40

116 Summers, Lawrence H., United States Government, statement to members of the African Development Bank, Abidjan, May 1993

117 OXFAM, op. cit., pp. 31-32

118 World Commission on Environment and Development (Brundtland Commission), op. cit.

119 United Nations, *Long-range World Population Projections: Two Centuries of Population Growth 1950-2150*, op. cit.

120 United Nations Children's Fund, *The Progress of Nations 1993*, op. cit., p. 35

121 See, for example, *Africa's Children, Africa's Future: Human Investment Priorities for the 1990s*, Organization of African Unity, Addis Ababa, and UNICEF, New York, 1992
See also United Nations Children's Fund, 'Debt Relief for Africa: A Call for Urgent Action on Human Development', UNICEF, New York, May 1993

122 *African Social and Economic Trends 1992*, Global Coalition for Africa, Washington, D.C., 1992

123 Food and Agriculture Organization of the United Nations, *The State of Food and Agriculture 1992*, FAO, Rome, 1992

124 *Africa's Children, Africa's Future: Human Investment Priorities for the 1990s*, op. cit., p. 7

125 United Nations Development Programme, *Human Development Report 1992*, op. cit., p.47

126 United Nations, 'African Debt Crisis: A Continuing Impediment to Development', United Nations, New York, 1993

127 OXFAM, op. cit.

128 Secretary-General of the United Nations, 'New Concepts of Development Action in Africa', SG/SM/4887, statement at United Nations, Geneva, December 1992

129 The 'Consensus of Dakar', providing a framework for African social development in accordance with the goals of the World Summit for Children, was adopted by the representatives of almost all African countries, 15 donor Governments, 5 international development agencies, and development banks and non-governmental organizations attending the Organization of African Unity International Conference on Assistance to African Children, Dakar, 25-27 November 1992

130 Secretary-General of the United Nations, 'Overcoming the Crisis in Development Cooperation', SG/SM/4872, statement to the Conference on Global Development Cooperation, Carter Center, Atlanta, 4 December 1992

131 Deger, Saadet, *The Economics of Disarmament: Prospects, Problems and Policies for the Disarmament Dividend*, op. cit.

132 'Consensus of Dakar', op. cit.

133 Quoted in 'Aid for Africa', *The Economist*, 14 May 1993

134 Quoted in Summers, Lawrence H., op. cit.

135 OXFAM, op. cit.

136 Gore, Al, op. cit., pp. 297-307

137 Sen, Amartya, *Poverty and Famines: An Essay on Entitlement and Deprivation*, Clarendon Press, Oxford, 1981

Statistical tables

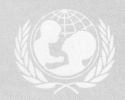

*Economic and social statistics on the nations of the world,
with particular reference to children's well-being.*

GENERAL NOTE ON THE DATA

The data provided in these tables are accompanied by definitions, sources, and explanations of symbols. Tables derived from so many sources – 12 major sources are listed in the explanatory material – will inevitably cover a wide range of data reliability. Official government data received by the responsible United Nations agency have been used whenever possible. In the many cases where there are no reliable official figures, estimates made by the responsible United Nations agency have been used. Where such internationally standardized estimates do not exist, the tables draw on other sources, particularly data received from the appropriate UNICEF field office. Where possible only comprehensive or representative national data have been used.

Data for life expectancy, crude birth and death rates, infant mortality rates, etc., are part of the regular work on estimates and projections undertaken by the United Nations Population Division. These and other internationally produced estimates are revised periodically, which explains why some of the data will differ from those found in earlier UNICEF publications. In particular, the under-five mortality rate (U5MR) estimates have been revised using new data and a methodology first applied on a small number of countries in the last report.

The recent creation of newly independent countries has resulted in 145 countries with populations of 1 million or more, instead of the 129 which were included in the previous report. In order to incorporate these new countries in the main tables, and still maintain easy readability, the regional summaries have been moved to a separate table (table 10).

Changes have been made to two indicators in this year's tables. One is a modification of 'still breastfeeding', from 12-15 months to 20-23 months. The prevalence of goitre in schoolchildren is the second inclusion. This indicator has been selected by UNICEF and WHO for monitoring iodine deficiency reduction, one of the goals of the World Summit for Children.

EXPLANATION OF SYMBOLS

Since the aim of the statistics section is to provide a broad picture of the situation of children and women worldwide, detailed data qualifications and footnotes are seen as more appropriate for inclusion elsewhere. Only two symbols are used in the tables.

.. Data not available

x Indicates data that refer to years or periods other than those specified in the column heading, differ from the standard definition, or refer to only part of a country.

U5MR estimates for individual countries are primarily derived from data reported by the United Nations Population Division. In some cases, these estimates may differ from the latest national figures. In general, data released during approximately the last year are not incorporated in these estimates.

INDEX TO COUNTRIES

In the following tables, countries are ranked in descending order of their estimated 1992 under-five mortality rate. The reference numbers indicating that rank are given in the alphabetical list of countries below.

Table 1: Basic indicators

#		Under-5 mortality rate		Infant mortality rate (under 1)		Total population (millions) 1992	Annual no. of births (thousands) 1992	Annual no. of under-5 deaths (thousands) 1992	GNP per capita (US$) 1991	Life expectancy at birth (years) 1992	Total adult literacy rate 1990	% of age-group enrolled in primary school (gross) 1986-1991	% share of household income 1980-1991	
		1960	1992	1960	1992								lowest 40%	highest 20%
1	Niger	320	**320**	191	191	8.3	428	137	300	46	28	29	. .	. .
2	Angola	345	**292**	208	170	9.9	514	150	610x	46	42	95	. .	. .
3	Mozambique	331	**287**	190	167	14.9	683	196	80	47	33	58	. .	. .
4	Afghanistan	360	**257**	215	165	19.1	1031	265	280x	43	29	24	. .	. .
5	Sierra Leone	385	**249**	219	144	4.4	213	53	210	43	21	48	. .	. .
6	Guinea-Bissau	336	**239**	200	141	1.0	43	10	180	43	37	59	. .	. .
7	Guinea	337	**230**	203	135	6.1	313	72	460	44	24	37	. .	. .
8	Malawi	365	**226**	206	143	10.4	567	128	230	44	. .	71	. .	. .
9	Rwanda	191	**222**	115	131	7.5	396	88	270	46	50	69	23	39
10	Mali	400	**220**	233	122	9.8	504	111	280	46	32	24	. .	. .
11	Liberia	288	**217**	192	146	2.8	132	29	450x	55	40	40x	. .	. .
12	Somalia	294	**211**	175	125	9.2	469	99	150x	47	24	15x	. .	. .
13	Chad	325	**209**	195	123	5.8	258	54	210	47	30	57	. .	. .
14	Eritrea	294	**208**	175	123	3.3	140	29	120	47	. .	. .	. .	. .
15	Ethiopia	294	**208**	175	123	53.0	2627	547	120	47	24x	38	21	41
16	Mauritania	321	**206**	191	118	2.1	100	21	510	48	34	51	40	. .
17	Zambia	220	**202**	135	113	8.6	403	81	420x	45	73	93	11x	61x
18	Bhutan	324	**201**	203	131	1.6	65	13	180	48	38	26	. .	. .
19	Nigeria	204	**191**	122	114	115.7	5259	1004	340	52	51	72	. .	. .
20	Zaire	286	**188**	167	121	39.9	1912	359	230x	52	72	78	. .	. .
21	Uganda	218	**185**	129	111	18.7	960	178	170	42	48	76	21	42
22	Cambodia	217	**184**	146	117	8.8	349	64	200x	51	35	. .	. .	. .
23	Burundi	255	**179**	151	108	5.8	271	48	210	48	50	72	. .	. .
24	Central African Rep.	294	**179**	174	105	3.2	142	25	390	47	38	67	. .	. .
25	Yemen	378	**177**	214	107	12.5	611	108	520	52	39	78	. .	. .
26	Tanzania, U. Rep. of	249	**176**	147	111	27.8	1351	238	100	51	. .	63	8	63
27	Ghana	215	**170**	128	103	16.0	671	114	400	56	60	75	18	44
28	Madagascar	364	**168**	219	110	12.8	589	99	210	55	80	92	. .	. .
29	Sudan	292	**166**	170	100	26.7	1128	187	420x	52	27	49	. .	. .
30	Gabon	287	**158**	171	95	1.2	53	8	3780	53	61	. .	. .	. .
31	Lesotho	204	**156**	138	108	1.8	64	10	580	60	. .	107	11	61
32	Burkina Faso	318	**150**	183	101	9.5	449	67	290	48	18	36	. .	. .
33	Benin	310	**147**	184	88	4.9	243	36	380	46	23	61	. .	. .
34	Senegal	303	**145**	174	90	7.7	334	48	720	49	38	58	. .	. .
35	Lao Peo. Dem. Rep.	233	**145**	155	98	4.5	205	30	220	51	84x	104	. .	. .
36	Pakistan	221	**137**	137	95	124.8	5117	701	400	59	35	37	21	40
37	Togo	264	**137**	155	86	3.8	169	23	410	55	43	103	. .	. .
38	Haiti	270	**133**	182	87	6.8	240	32	370	56	53	84	6x	48x
39	Nepal	279	**128**	186	90	20.6	778	100	180	53	26	86	22	40
40	Bangladesh	247	**127**	151	97	119.3	4623	587	220	53	35	73	23	39
41	Côte d'Ivoire	300	**124**	165	91	12.9	650	81	690	52	54	75x	19	42
42	India	236	**124**	144	83	879.5	25900	3212	330	60	48	97	21	41
43	Bolivia	252	**118**	152	80	7.5	261	31	650	61	78	82	12x	58x
44	Cameroon	264	**117**	156	74	12.2	499	58	850	56	54	101	. .	. .
45	Myanmar	237	**113**	158	83	43.7	1431	162	220x	57	81	127	. .	. .
46	Indonesia	216	**111**	127	71	191.2	5146	571	610	62	82	117	21	42
47	Congo	220	**110**	143	82	2.4	107	12	1120	52	57	. .	. .	. .
48	Libyan Arab Jamahiriya	269	**104**	160	70	4.9	206	21	5310x	63	64	. .	. .	. .
49	Turkmenistan	. .	**91**	. .	72	3.9	140	13	1700	66	. .	. .	23	. .
50	Turkey	217	**87**	161	70	58.4	1653	144	1780	67	81	110	11x	55x
51	Zimbabwe	181	**86**	109	60	10.6	434	37	650	56	67	117	. .	. .
52	Tajikistan	. .	**85**	. .	65	5.7	229	19	1050	69	. .	. .	23	. .
53	Iraq	171	**80**	117	64	19.3	753	60	1500x	66	60	96	. .	. .
54	Mongolia	185	**80**	128	61	2.3	79	6	780x	63	. .	98	. .	. .
55	Namibia	206	**79**	129	62	1.5	66	5	1460	58	. .	94	. .	. .
56	Papua New Guinea	248	**77**	165	54	4.1	136	11	830	56	52	71	. .	. .
57	Guatemala	205	**76**	137	55	9.7	380	29	930	64	55	77	8	63
58	Nicaragua	209	**76**	140	54	4.0	163	12	460	66	. .	98	12x	58x
59	Kenya	202	**74**	120	51	25.2	1111	82	340	59	69	94	9	61
60	Algeria	243	**72**	148	60	26.3	901	65	1980	66	57	95	. .	. .
61	South Africa	126	**70**	89	53	39.8	1253	88	2560	63	76x	. .	. .	. .
62	Uzbekistan	. .	**68**	. .	56	21.5	736	50	1350	69	. .	. .	22	. .
63	Brazil	181	**65**	118	54	154.1	3626	236	2940	66	81	108x	7	68
64	Peru	236	**65**	143	46	22.5	658	43	1070	64	85	126	14	51
65	El Salvador	210	**63**	130	47	5.4	182	11	1080	66	73	78	8x	66x
66	Morocco	215	**61**	133	50	26.3	854	52	1030	63	50	68	17	46
67	Kyrgyzstan	. .	**60**	. .	49	4.5	135	8	1550	66	. .	. .	21	. .
68	Philippines	102	**60**	73	46	65.2	1992	120	730	65	90	111	17	48
69	Ecuador	180	**59**	115	47	11.1	332	20	1000	66	86	118	. .	. .
70	Botswana	170	**58**	117	45	1.3	51	3	2530	61	74	110	6	66
71	Honduras	203	**58**	137	45	5.5	205	12	580	66	73	108	9	64
72	Iran, Islamic Rep. of	233	**58**	145	44	61.6	2473	143	2170	67	54	112	. .	. .
73	Egypt	258	**55**	169	43	54.8	1732	95	610	61	48	98	21x	41x
74	Azerbaijan	. .	**53**	. .	37	7.3	189	10	1670	71	. .	. .	. .	. .
75	Dominican Rep.	152	**50**	104	42	7.5	214	11	940	67	83	95	12	56

		Under-5 mortality rate		Infant mortality rate (under 1)		Total population (millions)	Annual no. of births (thousands)	Annual no. of under-5 deaths (thousands)	GNP per capita (US$)	Life expectancy at birth (years)	Total adult literacy rate	% of age-group enrolled in primary school Total	% share of household income 1980-1991	
		1960	1992	1960	1992	1992	1992	1992	1991	1992	1990	1986-1991	lowest 40%	highest 20%
76	Kazakhstan	..	**50**	..	43	17.0	351	18	2470	69	..	..	..	..
77	Viet Nam	219	**49**	147	37	69.5	2039	100	240x	64	88	102x	..	..
78	Lebanon	91	**44**	68	35	2.8	78	3	2150x	68	80	100x	..	..
79	China	209	**43**	140	35	1188.0	25057	1077	370	71	73	135	17	42
80	Saudi Arabia	292	**40**	170	35	15.9	574	23	7820	69	62	78	..	..
81	Syrian Arab Rep.	201	**40**	136	34	13.3	569	23	1160	67	65	109	..	..
82	Tunisia	244	**38**	163	32	8.4	230	9	1500	68	65	116	16	46
83	Moldova	..	**36**	..	31	4.4	69	2	2170	68	..	..	23	..
84	Albania	151	**34**	112	28	3.3	76	3	790x	73	..	98	..	..
85	Armenia	..	**34**	..	29	3.5	79	3	2150	72	..	..	22	..
86	Paraguay	90	**34**	66	28	4.5	151	5	1270	67	90	107	..	..
87	Korea, Dem. Peo. Rep.	120	**33**	85	25	22.6	553	18	970x	71	..	106	..	..
88	Mexico	141	**33**	98	28	88.2	2491	82	3030	70	88	112	12	56
89	Thailand	146	**33**	101	27	56.1	1176	39	1570	69	93	85	16	51
90	Russian Federation	..	**32**	..	28	148.3	1809	58	3220	69	..	..	..	..
91	Oman	300	**31**	180	24	1.6	67	2	6120	69	..	103	..	..
92	Jordan	149	**30**	103	25	4.3	171	5	1050	68	80	104x	..	..
93	Georgia	..	**29**	..	25	5.5	84	2	1640	73	..	..	21	..
94	Romania	82	**28**	69	23	23.3	363	10	1390	70	..	91	..	..
95	Latvia	..	**26**	..	22	2.7	37	1	3410	71	..	..	..	..
96	Ukraine	..	**25**	..	21	51.9	633	16	2340	70	..	..	21	..
97	Argentina	68	**24**	57	22	33.1	673	16	2790	71	95	111	14x	51x
98	Estonia	..	**24**	..	20	1.6	22	1	3830	71	100x	..	20	..
99	Mauritius	84	**24**	62	20	1.1	20	0	2410	70	..	106	12x	46x
100	Venezuela	70	**24**	53	20	20.2	531	13	2730x	70	88	92	14	50
101	Belarus	..	**23**	..	20	10.3	136	3	3110	71	..	..	22	..
102	Trinidad and Tobago	73	**22**	61	19	1.3	30	1	3670	71	95x	95	13x	50x
103	United Arab Emirates	240	**22**	160	18	1.7	35	1	19860x	71	..	116	..	..
104	Uruguay	47	**22**	41	20	3.1	54	1	2840	72	96	106	18x	44x
105	Yugoslavia (former)	113	**22**	92	19	23.9	338	7	3060x	72	93	95	16	44
106	Colombia	132	**20**	82	17	33.4	809	16	1260	69	87	110	13	53
107	Lithuania	..	**20**	..	17	3.8	56	1	2710	73	98x	..	..	..
108	Panama	104	**20**	67	18	2.5	63	1	2130	73	88	107	8	60
109	Bulgaria	70	**20**	49	16	9.0	111	2	1840	72	..	96	..	..
110	Sri Lanka	130	**19**	90	15	17.7	371	7	500	71	88	107	13	56
111	Malaysia	105	**19**	73	14	18.8	545	10	2520	71	78	93	13	54
112	Chile	138	**18**	107	15	13.6	309	6	2160	72	93	98	11	63
113	Kuwait	128	**17**	89	14	2.0	54	1	16150x	75	73	100	..	..
114	Poland	70	**16**	62	14	38.4	550	9	1790	72	..	98	23	36
115	Hungary	57	**16**	51	15	10.5	127	2	2720	70	99x	94	26	34
116	Costa Rica	112	**16**	80	14	3.2	85	1	1850	76	93	102	13	51
117	Jamaica	76	**14**	58	12	2.5	55	1	1380	73	98	105	16	48
118	Slovakia	..	**14**	..	12	5.4	79	1	..	72	..	..	..	..
119	Portugal	112	**13**	81	11	9.9	114	2	5930	75	85	119	..	..
120	Czech Republic	..	**12**	..	11	10.4	135	2	..	72	..	..	..	..
121	Cuba	50	**11**	39	10	10.8	190	2	1170x	76	94	103	..	..
122	Israel	39	**11**	32	9	5.1	110	1	11950	76	92x	93	18	40
123	Belgium	35	**11**	31	9	10.0	122	1	18950	76	..	102	22	36
124	USA	30	**10**	26	9	255.2	4078	42	22240	76	..	105	16	42
125	New Zealand	26	**10**	22	8	3.5	60	1	12350	76	..	106	16	45
126	Italy	50	**10**	44	8	57.8	578	6	18520	77	97	97	19	41
127	Spain	57	**9**	46	8	39.1	422	4	12450	77	95	109	19	40
128	Greece	64	**9**	53	8	10.2	106	1	6340	77	93	100	..	..
129	Korea, Rep. of	124	**9**	88	8	44.2	723	7	6330	71	96	107	20x	42x
130	Austria	43	**9**	37	7	7.8	91	1	20140	76	..	103	..	..
131	France	34	**9**	29	7	57.2	773	7	20380	77	..	111	18	41
132	United Kingdom	27	**9**	23	7	57.7	801	7	16550	76	..	107	17	40
133	Australia	24	**9**	20	7	17.6	265	2	17050	77	..	105	16	42
134	Switzerland	27	**9**	22	7	6.8	86	1	33610	78	..	..	17	45
135	Germany	40	**8**	34	7	80.3	912	8	23650	76	..	105	20	39
136	Canada	33	**8**	28	7	27.4	391	3	20440	77	..	105	18	40
137	Denmark	25	**8**	22	7	5.2	64	1	23700	76	..	98	17	39
138	Norway	23	**8**	19	6	4.3	63	0	24220	77	..	99	19	37
139	Netherlands	22	**7**	18	6	15.2	207	2	18780	77	..	117	20	38
140	Sweden	20	**7**	16	6	8.7	120	1	25110	78	..	107	21	37
141	Hong Kong	52	**7**	38	6	5.8	75	1	13430	78	..	105	16	47
142	Singapore	40	**7**	31	6	2.8	44	0	14210	74	83x	110	15	49
143	Finland	28	**7**	22	6	5.0	64	0	23980	76	..	99	18	38
144	Japan	40	**6**	31	4	124.5	1390	8	26930	79	..	101	22	38
145	Ireland	36	**6**	31	5	3.5	50	0	11120	75	..	100	..	..

Countries listed in descending order of their under-five mortality rates (shown in bold type).

Table 2: Nutrition

#		% of infants with low birth weight 1990	% of children (1986-92) who are:			% of children (1980-92) suffering from:				Total goitre rate (6-11 years) (%) 1980-92	Daily per capita calorie supply as a % of requirements 1988-90	% share of total household consumption (1980-85)	
			exclusively breastfed (0-3 months)	breastfed with complementary food (6-9 months)	still breastfeeding (20-23 months)	underweight (0-4 years) moderate & severe	severe	wasting (12-23 months) moderate & severe	stunting (24-59 months) moderate & severe			all food	cereals
1	Niger	15	..	..	..	49	..	23x	38x	9	95	..	..
2	Angola	19	3	83	53	..	..	..	..	7	80	..	..
3	Mozambique	20	..	..	..	..	..	..	..	20	77	..	..
4	Afghanistan	20	..	..	..	..	..	..	..	20	72	..	..
5	Sierra Leone	17	..	94	41	29	..	18	39	7	83	56	22
6	Guinea-Bissau	20	..	..	..	23x	..	..	..	19	97	..	..
7	Guinea	21	..	..	..	..	..	..	..	19	97	..	..
8	Malawi	20	3	89	..	27	8	11	62	13	88	30	9
9	Rwanda	17	90	75	..	29x	6x	9x	58x	49	82	29	10
10	Mali	17	8	45	44	31x	9x	16	34x	29	96	57	22
11	Liberia	..	15	56	26	20x	..	..	..	6	98	..	..
12	Somalia	16	..	..	..	..	..	..	..	7	81	..	..
13	Chad	..	..	..	..	..	..	..	..	15	73	..	..
14	Eritrea	..	..	..	..	..	..	..	..	..	..	..	..
15	Ethiopia	16	74	..	35	48x	16x	12x	63x	22	73	49	24
16	Mauritania	11	12	39	..	48	..	18	65	..	106	..	..
17	Zambia	13	13	88	34	25	6	10	47	51x	87	36	8
18	Bhutan	..	..	..	..	38	..	4x	56x	25	128	..	..
19	Nigeria	16	2	52	43	36	12	16	54	10	93	48	18
20	Zaire	15	..	..	..	..	..	..	..	9	96	..	..
21	Uganda	..	70	67	39	23x	5x	4x	51x	7	93	..	..
22	Cambodia	..	..	..	..	..	..	..	..	15	96	..	..
23	Burundi	..	89	66	73	38x	10x	10	60x	42	84	..	..
24	Central African Rep.	15	..	..	..	..	..	..	..	63	82	..	..
25	Yemen	19	15	51	..	30	4	17	49	32	..	..	..
26	Tanzania, U. Rep. of	14	32	59	57	29	7	10	58	37	95	64	32
27	Ghana	17	2	57	52	27	6	15	39	10	93	50	..
28	Madagascar	10	..	..	..	33x	8x	17	56x	24	95	59	26
29	Sudan	15	14	45	44	35x	7x	13x	32x	20	87	60	..
30	Gabon	..	..	..	..	..	..	..	..	5	104	..	..
31	Lesotho	11	..	..	..	16	2	7	23	16	93	..	..
32	Burkina Faso	21x	3	35	..	..	..	..	..	16	94	..	..
33	Benin	..	..	..	..	..	..	..	..	24	104	37	12
34	Senegal	11	7	68	37	22	2	8	30	12	98	49	15
35	Lao Peo. Dem. Rep.	18	..	..	..	37	..	20	44	25	111	..	..
36	Pakistan	25	25	29	52	40	14	11	60	32	99	37	12
37	Togo	20	10	86	68	24x	6x	10	37x	22	99	..	..
38	Haiti	15	..	..	..	37x	3x	17x	51x	4x	89	..	..
39	Nepal	..	..	..	..	..	..	..	..	44	100	57	38
40	Bangladesh	50	..	..	..	66	27	28	65	11	88	59	36
41	Côte d'Ivoire	14x	..	..	..	12	2	17	20	6	111	39	13
42	India	33	..	..	..	63x	27x	..	65x	9	101	52	18
43	Bolivia	12	59	57	30	13x	3x	2	51x	21	84	33	..
44	Cameroon	13	7	77	35	14	3	7	32	26	95	24	7
45	Myanmar	16	..	..	..	32x	9x	..	..	18	114	..	..
46	Indonesia	14	53	76	62	40	..	..	..	28	121	48	21
47	Congo	16	43	..	27	24	..	13	33	8	103	37	16
48	Libyan Arab Jamahiriya	..	..	..	..	..	..	..	..	6	140	..	..
49	Turkmenistan	..	..	..	..	..	..	..	..	20	..	..	..
50	Turkey	8	..	..	..	..	..	..	..	36	127	40	9
51	Zimbabwe	14	11	94	26	12	2	2	31	42	94	40	9
52	Tajikistan	..	..	..	..	..	..	..	..	20	..	..	..
53	Iraq	15	..	..	..	12	2	..	..	7	128	..	..
54	Mongolia	10	..	..	..	12x	..	2x	29x	7	97	..	..
55	Namibia	12	22	65	23	26	6	13	29	35	..	..	..
56	Papua New Guinea	23	..	..	..	35	..	..	..	30	114	..	..
57	Guatemala	14	..	..	44	34x	8x	3	68x	20	103	36	10
58	Nicaragua	15	..	..	..	11	1	0	22	4	99	..	..
59	Kenya	16	24	87	46	14x	3x	5x	32x	7	89	38	16
60	Algeria	9	..	..	..	9	..	7	18	9	123	..	..
61	South Africa	..	..	..	..	..	..	..	..	2	128	34	..
62	Uzbekistan	..	..	..	..	..	..	..	..	18	..	..	..
63	Brazil	11	4	27	13	7	1	3	16	14x	114	35	9
64	Peru	11	40	62	36	11	2	3	46	36	87	35	8
65	El Salvador	11	..	..	..	15	..	3	36	25	102	33	12
66	Morocco	9	48	48	18	16x	4x	6	34x	20	125	38	12
67	Kyrgyzstan	..	..	..	..	..	..	..	..	20	..	..	..
68	Philippines	15	..	..	..	34	5	14	45	15	104	51	21
69	Ecuador	11	31	31	23	17	0	4	39	10	105	30	..
70	Botswana	8	41	82	23	15x	..	..	..	8	97	25	12
71	Honduras	9	..	..	..	21	4	2x	34x	9	98	39	..
72	Iran, Islamic Rep. of	9	..	..	..	..	..	..	..	30	125	37	10
73	Egypt	10	38	52	..	10	3	4	32	5	132	49	10
74	Azerbaijan	..	..	..	..	..	..	..	..	20	..	..	..
75	Dominican Rep.	16	10	23	7	10	2	1	22	..	102	46	13

No.	Country	% of infants with low birth weight 1990	% of children (1986-92) who are: exclusively breastfed (0-3 months)	breastfed with complementary food (6-9 months)	still breastfeeding (20-23 months)	% of children (1980-92) suffering from: underweight (0-4 years) moderate & severe	underweight severe	wasting (12-23 months) moderate & severe	stunting (24-59 months) moderate & severe	Total goitre rate (6-11 years) (%) 1980-92	Daily per capita calorie supply as a % of requirements 1988-90	% share of total household consumption (1980-85) all food	cereals
76	Kazakhstan	..	..	..	..	..	..	..	..	20	..	..	..
77	Viet Nam	17	..	..	..	42	14	12x	49x	20	103	..	..
78	Lebanon	10	..	..	..	..	..	..	..	15	127	..	..
79	China	9	..	..	..	21x	3x	8x	41x	9	112	61	..
80	Saudi Arabia	7	..	..	..	..	..	..	..	..	121	..	..
81	Syrian Arab Rep.	11	..	..	..	..	..	..	..	73	126	..	..
82	Tunisia	8	21	53	25	10x	2x	4	23x	4	131	37	7
83	Moldova	..	..	..	..	..	..	..	..	..	..	..	..
84	Albania	7	..	..	..	..	..	..	..	41	107	..	..
85	Armenia	..	..	..	..	..	..	..	..	10	..	..	..
86	Paraguay	8	7	61	8	4	1	0	17	49	116	30	6
87	Korea, Dem. Peo. Rep.	..	..	..	..	..	..	..	..	..	121	..	..
88	Mexico	12	37	36	21	14	..	6x	22x	15	131	35	..
89	Thailand	13	4	69	34	26x	4x	10	28x	12	103	30	7
90	Russian Federation	..	..	..	..	..	..	..	..	..	..	..	..
91	Oman	10	..	..	..	23	5	11	22	..	..	..	..
92	Jordan	7	32	48	13	6	1	3	21	..	110	35	..
93	Georgia	..	..	..	..	..	..	..	..	20	..	..	..
94	Romania	7	..	..	..	..	..	..	..	10	116	..	..
95	Latvia	..	..	..	..	..	..	..	..	..	..	..	..
96	Ukraine	..	..	..	..	..	..	..	..	10	..	..	..
97	Argentina	8	..	..	..	..	..	..	..	8	131	35	4
98	Estonia	..	..	..	..	..	..	..	..	..	..	..	..
99	Mauritius	9	..	..	..	24	..	16x	22x	..	128	24	7
100	Venezuela	9	..	..	..	6	..	4	7	11	99	23	..
101	Belarus	..	..	..	..	..	..	..	..	22	..	..	..
102	Trinidad and Tobago	10	10	39	16	7x	0x	5	4x	..	114	19	3
103	United Arab Emirates	6	..	..	26	..	..	..	..	..	..	..	..
104	Uruguay	8	..	..	..	7x	2x	..	16x	..	101	31	7
105	Yugoslavia (former)	..	..	..	..	..	..	..	..	5	140	27	4
106	Colombia	10	17	48	24	10x	2x	5	18x	10	106	29	..
107	Lithuania	..	..	..	..	..	..	..	..	..	..	..	..
108	Panama	10	..	..	..	16	..	7	24	13	98	38	7
109	Bulgaria	6	..	..	..	..	..	..	..	20	148	..	..
110	Sri Lanka	25	14	47	46	29x	2x	21x	39x	14	101	43	18
111	Malaysia	10	..	..	..	..	..	..	..	20	120	23	..
112	Chile	7	..	..	..	3x	0x	1	10x	9	102	29	7
113	Kuwait	7	..	..	..	6	..	2	14	..	..	..	..
114	Poland	..	..	..	..	..	..	..	..	10	131	29	4
115	Hungary	9	..	..	..	..	..	..	..	..	137	25	3
116	Costa Rica	6	..	..	..	6	..	3	8	3	121	33	8
117	Jamaica	11	..	..	..	7	1	6	7	..	114	36	14
118	Slovakia	..	..	..	..	..	..	..	..	..	..	..	..
119	Portugal	5	..	..	..	..	..	..	..	15	136	34	8
120	Czech Republic	..	..	..	..	..	..	..	..	..	..	..	..
121	Cuba	8	..	..	..	..	..	1x	..	10	135	..	..
122	Israel	7	..	..	..	..	..	..	..	..	125	21	..
123	Belgium	6	..	..	..	..	..	..	..	5	149	15	2
124	USA	7	..	..	..	..	..	..	..	..	138	10	2
125	New Zealand	6	..	..	..	..	..	..	..	..	131	12	2
126	Italy	5	..	..	..	..	..	..	..	20	139	19	2
127	Spain	4	..	..	..	..	..	..	..	10	141	24	3
128	Greece	6	..	..	..	..	..	..	..	10	151	30	3
129	Korea, Rep. of	9	..	..	..	..	..	..	..	..	120	35	14
130	Austria	6	..	..	..	..	..	..	..	..	133	16	2
131	France	5	..	..	..	..	..	..	..	5	143	16	2
132	United Kingdom	7	..	..	..	..	..	..	..	..	130	12	2
133	Australia	6	..	..	..	..	..	..	..	..	124	13	2
134	Switzerland	5	..	..	..	..	..	..	..	..	130	17	..
135	Germany	..	..	..	..	..	..	..	..	10	..	12	2
136	Canada	6	..	..	..	..	..	..	..	..	122	11	2
137	Denmark	6	..	..	..	..	..	..	..	5	135	13	2
138	Norway	4	..	..	..	..	..	..	..	..	120	15	2
139	Netherlands	..	..	..	..	..	..	..	..	3	114	13	2
140	Sweden	5	..	..	..	..	..	..	..	..	111	13	2
141	Hong Kong	8	..	..	..	..	..	..	..	..	125	12	1
142	Singapore	7	..	..	..	14x	..	..	..	..	136	19	..
143	Finland	4	..	..	..	..	..	..	..	..	113	16	3
144	Japan	6	..	..	..	..	..	..	..	..	125	17	4
145	Ireland	4	..	..	..	..	..	..	..	..	157	22	4

Countries listed in descending order of their 1992 under-five mortality rates (table 1).

Table 3: Health

#	Country	Safe water total	Safe water urban	Safe water rural	Sanitation total	Sanitation urban	Sanitation rural	Health total	Health urban	Health rural	TB	DPT	polio	measles	pregnant women tetanus	ORT use rate 1987-92
		| % of population with access to safe water 1988-91			% of population with access to adequate sanitation 1988-91			% of population with access to health services 1985-92			% fully immunized 1990-92 — 1-year-old children					
1	Niger	53	98	45	14	71	4	41	99	30	40	21	21	28	45	17
2	Angola	41	71	20	19	25	15	30x	..	..	27	12	13	26	8	48
3	Mozambique	22	44	17	20	61	11	39	100	30	64	53	53	60	32	30
4	Afghanistan	23	40	19	..	13	..	29	80	17	48	27	27	37	9	26
5	Sierra Leone	37	33	37	58	92	49	38	90	20	89	72	72	65	80	60
6	Guinea-Bissau	41	56	35	31	27	32	..	..	..	100	66	65	60	35	6
7	Guinea	53	87	56	21	84	5	75	100	55	65	52	52	50	70	65
8	Malawi	56x	97x	50x	84	100	81	80	..	..	99	86	84	82	66	14
9	Rwanda	66	75	62	58	77	56	80	..	..	94	85	85	81	88	26
10	Mali	41	53	38	24	81	10	35	..	..	70	34	34	41	8	41
11	Liberia	50	93	22	..	..	..	39	50	30	78	28	28	61	20	15
12	Somalia	37	50	29	18	44	5	27x	50x	15x	31x	18x	18x	30x	5x	78
13	Chad	57	25	70	..	..	..	30	..	..	43	17	17	41	5	15
14	Eritrea	..	..	..	..	..	..	..	..	..	..	..	..	..	..	..
15	Ethiopia	25	91	19	19	97	7	46	..	..	21	13	13	10	7	68
16	Mauritania	66	67	65	..	34	..	45	72	33	73	34	34	39	40	54
17	Zambia	53	70	28	37	75	12	75x	100x	50x	83	57	59	56	20	90
18	Bhutan	34	60	30	13	50	7	65	..	..	81	79	77	82	43	85
19	Nigeria	36	81	30	35	40	30	66	85	62	50	31	30	36	25	80
20	Zaire	39	68	24	23	46	11	26	40	17	65x	32x	31x	31x	29x	45
21	Uganda	33	60	30	32	63	28	61x	90x	57x	98	72	72	70	16	30
22	Cambodia	36	65	33	14	81	8	53	80	50	50	32	32	33	22	6
23	Burundi	57	99	54	49	71	47	80	100	79	91	80	80	70	56	49
24	Central African Rep.	24	19	26	46	45	46	45	..	..	94	77	77	62	87	24
25	Yemen	36	61	30	65	87	60	38	81	32	77	62	62	64	13	6
26	Tanzania, U. Rep. of	49	65	45	64	74	62	76x	99x	72x	99	84	83	82	15	83
27	Ghana	52	93	35	42	64	32	60	92	45	57	34	36	40	9	44
28	Madagascar	23	55	9	3	12	3	65	65	65	46	32	32	27	2	29
29	Sudan	48	55	43	75	89	65	51	90	40	75	67	67	66	14	28
30	Gabon	68	90	50	..	..	..	90x	..	..	96	78	78	76	86	25
31	Lesotho	47	59	45	22	14	23	80	..	..	59	58	58	80	40	78
32	Burkina Faso	68	44	72	10	35	5	49x	51x	48x	66	39	39	41	26	15
33	Benin	51	66	46	34	42	31	18	..	..	84	73	73	70	83	45
34	Senegal	48	84	26	55	85	36	40	..	..	65	47	47	43	26	27
35	Lao Peo. Dem. Rep.	36	54	33	21	97	8	67	..	..	39	23	25	55	19	30
36	Pakistan	56	80	45	24	55	10	55	99	35	91	78	78	76	42	34
37	Togo	60	77	53	23	56	10	61	..	..	74	53	47	29	81	33
38	Haiti	39	55	33	24	55	16	50	..	..	45	24	27	24	5	20
39	Nepal	42	67	39	6	52	3	..	..	..	82	72	72	64	18	14
40	Bangladesh	84	82	81	31	63	26	45	..	..	89	63	63	59	80	24
41	Côte d'Ivoire	76	70	81	60	59	62	30x	61x	11x	47	47	47	51	35	16
42	India	85	87	85	16	53	2	..	..	..	96	89	89	85	77	37
43	Bolivia	52	77	27	26	40	13	63	90	36	86	77	84	80	52	63
44	Cameroon	48	100	27	74	100	64	41	44	39	52	37	37	37	7	84
45	Myanmar	32	37	..	36	39	35	48	..	..	80	73	73	71	72	19
46	Indonesia	51	68	43	44	64	36	80	..	..	95	91	91	89	60	44
47	Congo	38	92	2	..	..	..	83	97	70	88	74	74	64	60	67
48	Libyan Arab Jamahiriya	97	100	80	98	100	85	..	..	..	91	62	62	59	16	80
49	Turkmenistan	..	..	..	..	..	..	..	..	..	97	84	91	76	..	..
50	Turkey	78x	95x	63x	..	..	..	..	..	..	65	76	76	72	22	..
51	Zimbabwe	84	95	80	40	95	22	85	96	80	79	73	73	72	60	77
52	Tajikistan	..	..	..	..	..	..	..	..	..	..	92	..	..	..	..
53	Iraq	77	93	41	..	96	..	93	97	78	79	63	64	68	45	70
54	Mongolia	80	100	58	74	100	47	95	..	..	85	84	84	86	..	65
55	Namibia	52	98	35	14	24	11	72	92	60	90	65	65	63	52	..
56	Papua New Guinea	33	94	20	..	57	..	96	..	..	67	61	61	66	52	46
57	Guatemala	62	92	43	60	72	52	34	47	25	56	65	69	58	18	24
58	Nicaragua	54	76	21	..	78	..	83	100	60	79	73	86	72	12	40
59	Kenya	49	74	43	43	69	35	77	..	40	93	85	85	81	37	69
60	Algeria	68x	85x	55x	57	80	40	88	100	80	97	89	89	82	27	27
61	South Africa	..	..	..	..	..	..	..	..	..	85	67	69	63	..	..
62	Uzbekistan	..	95	61	..	..	32	..	..	..	97	63	85	84	..	..
63	Brazil	87	95	61	72	84	32	..	..	..	87	69	62	93	21	63
64	Peru	56	77	10	57	77	20	75x	..	..	82	80	81	80	27	31
65	El Salvador	47	85	19	58	86	36	56	80	40	71	65	65	62	26	45
66	Morocco	56	100	18	..	100	..	70	100	50	93	87	81	81	80	13
67	Kyrgyzstan	..	..	..	..	..	..	..	..	..	96	88	91	94	..	..
68	Philippines	82	85	79	69	78	62	75	77	74	94	92	92	90	52	25
69	Ecuador	55	63	43	48	56	38	88	..	..	99	83	83	66	5	70
70	Botswana	90	100	88	88	100	85	89x	100x	85x	71	82	82	65	46	64
71	Honduras	77	98	63	61	98	43	66	80	56	91	93	95	89	16	70
72	Iran, Islamic Rep. of	89	100	75	71	100	35	80	95	65	92	87	87	84	87	85
73	Egypt	90	95	86	50	80	26	..	..	..	92	89	89	89	70	34
74	Azerbaijan	..	..	..	..	..	..	..	..	..	53	69	70	50	..	..
75	Dominican Rep.	67	82	45	87	95	75	80	..	..	48	48	63	75	24	35

No.	Country	% of population with access to safe water 1988-91			% of population with access to adequate sanitation 1988-91			% of population with access to health services 1985-92			% fully immunized 1990-92 1-year-old children				pregnant women tetanus	ORT use rate 1987-92
		total	urban	rural	total	urban	rural	total	urban	rural	TB	DPT	polio	measles		
76	Kazakhstan	..	..	..	..	..	..	..	..	..	90	85	87	90	..	..
77	Viet Nam	24	39	21	17	34	13	91	100	80	91	88	89	90	42	52
78	Lebanon	92	95	85	..	..	..	95	98	85	4	85	85	51	..	45
79	China	72	87	68	79	68	81	90	100	88	94	94	95	94	3	22
80	Saudi Arabia	95	100	74	86	100	30	97	100	88	97	96	96	90	62	45
81	Syrian Arab Rep.	74	90	58	83	84	82	83	92	68	93	89	89	84	63	95
82	Tunisia	99	100	99	96	98	94	90x	100x	80x	80	95	95	87	44	22
83	Moldova	..	..	..	..	..	..	..	..	..	96	89	93	92	..	..
84	Albania	..	..	..	..	..	..	..	..	..	94	94	96	87	..	..
85	Armenia	..	..	..	..	..	..	..	..	..	..	..	..	..	..	..
86	Paraguay	35	50	24	62	56	67	61	..	..	99	85	87	86	54	52
87	Korea, Dem. Peo. Rep.	..	..	..	..	..	..	..	..	..	99	90	98	96	97	72
88	Mexico	76	81	68	50	70	17	78	80	60	95	91	92	91	42	63
89	Thailand	77	87	72	74	80	72	90	90	90	99	85	84	74	72	65
90	Russian Federation	..	..	..	..	..	..	..	..	..	88	73	69	83	..	..
91	Oman	84	91	77	71	75	40	95	100	95	97	97	97	97	97	19
92	Jordan	99	100	97	100	100	100	97	98	95	..	98	97	91	32	77
93	Georgia	..	..	..	..	..	..	..	..	..	63	45	45	58	..	..
94	Romania	..	..	..	..	..	..	..	..	..	99	97	90	92	..	..
95	Latvia	..	..	..	..	..	..	..	..	..	94	87	92	95	..	..
96	Ukraine	..	..	..	..	..	..	..	..	..	93	88	89	90	..	..
97	Argentina	65	73	17	69	75	35	71	80	21	99	78	83	89	..	70
98	Estonia	..	..	..	..	..	..	..	..	..	96	70	71	75	..	..
99	Mauritius	96	100	92	94	92	96	100	100	100	87	91	91	87	77	7
100	Venezuela	89	89	89	92	97	70	..	..	..	82	66	72	61	..	80
101	Belarus	..	..	..	..	..	..	..	..	..	94	90	90	94	..	..
102	Trinidad and Tobago	97	99	91	79	99	98	99	..	..	..	82	81	93	..	70
103	United Arab Emirates	95	..	..	77	93	22	99	..	..	98	86	86	85	..	81
104	Uruguay	75	85	5	61	60	65	82	..	..	99	93	93	93	13	96
105	Yugoslavia (former)	..	..	..	..	..	..	..	..	..	81	79	81	76	..	..
106	Colombia	86	87	82	64	84	18	60	..	..	86	77	84	74	40	40
107	Lithuania	..	..	..	..	..	..	..	..	..	94	78	88	89	..	..
108	Panama	83	100	66	84	100	68	80x	95x	64x	98	82	83	71	27	55
109	Bulgaria	..	..	..	..	..	..	..	..	..	100	99	99	97	..	..
110	Sri Lanka	60	80	55	50	68	45	93x	..	..	89	86	86	79	67	76
111	Malaysia	78	96	66	81	..	..	..	..	..	99	90	90	79	83	47
112	Chile	86	100	..	83	100	20	97	..	..	99	91	91	90	..	10
113	Kuwait	..	100	..	..	100	..	100	..	..	3	92	92	93	22	10
114	Poland	..	..	..	..	..	..	..	..	..	94	98	98	94	..	..
115	Hungary	..	..	..	..	..	..	..	..	..	99	100	98	100	..	..
116	Costa Rica	93	100	86	97	100	94	80x	100x	63x	92	90	90	84	68	78
117	Jamaica	100	100	100	89	100	80	90	..	..	85	84	74	63	50	10
118	Slovakia	..	..	..	..	..	..	..	..	..	91	99	99	96	..	..
119	Portugal	..	..	..	..	..	..	..	..	..	89	95	95	96	..	..
120	Czech Republic	..	..	..	..	..	..	..	..	..	98	99	99	97	..	..
121	Cuba	98	100	91	92	100	68	98	99	96	98	91	93	98	98	80
122	Israel	..	..	..	..	..	..	..	..	..	..	85x	89x	88x	..	..
123	Belgium	..	..	..	..	..	..	..	..	..	..	87	99	75	..	..
124	USA	..	..	..	..	..	..	..	..	..	..	58	74	77	..	..
125	New Zealand	97	100	82	..	..	..	..	..	..	20	81	68	82	..	..
126	Italy	..	..	..	..	..	..	..	..	..	6	95	85	50	..	..
127	Spain	..	..	..	..	..	..	..	..	..	..	93	94	97	..	..
128	Greece	..	..	..	..	..	..	..	..	..	56	54	96	76	..	..
129	Korea, Rep. of	97	97	96	100	100	100	100	100	100	76	80	79	96	..	..
130	Austria	..	..	..	..	..	..	..	..	..	97	90	90	60	..	..
131	France	..	..	..	..	..	..	..	..	..	80	95	85	71	..	..
132	United Kingdom	..	..	..	..	..	..	..	..	..	75	90	95	89	..	..
133	Australia	..	..	..	..	..	..	..	..	..	..	95	72	86	..	..
134	Switzerland	..	..	..	..	..	..	..	..	..	..	89	95	83	..	..
135	Germany	..	..	..	..	..	..	..	..	..	84	95	95	80	..	..
136	Canada	..	..	..	..	..	..	..	..	..	85x	85x	70x	85x	..	..
137	Denmark	..	..	..	..	..	..	..	..	..	..	99	99	86	..	..
138	Norway	..	..	..	..	..	..	..	..	..	95	91	86	90	..	..
139	Netherlands	..	..	..	..	..	..	..	..	..	..	97	97	94	..	..
140	Sweden	..	..	..	..	..	..	..	..	..	14	99	99	95	..	..
141	Hong Kong	100	100	96	88	90	50	99x	..	..	94	90	90	42	..	..
142	Singapore	100	100	..	99	99	..	100	100	..	99	85	85	90	..	..
143	Finland	..	..	..	..	..	..	..	..	..	99	95	97	97	..	..
144	Japan	97	100	85	..	85	..	..	..	..	85	87	90	66	..	..
145	Ireland	..	..	..	..	..	..	..	..	..	..	65	81	78	..	..

Countries listed in descending order of their 1992 under-five mortality rates (table 1).

Table 4: Education

		Adult literacy rate 1970		Adult literacy rate 1990		No. of sets per 1000 population 1990		Primary school enrolment ratio 1960 (gross)		Primary school enrolment ratio 1986-91 (gross)		Primary school enrolment ratio 1986-91 (net)		% of grade 1 enrolment reaching final grade of primary school 1988	Secondary school enrolment ratio 1986-91 (gross)	
		male	female	male	female	radio	television	male	female	male	female	male	female		male	female
1	Niger	6	2	40	17	60	5	8	3	37	21	31	19	75	9	4
2	Angola	16	7	56	29	54	6	30	14	98	91	..	..	..	..	..
3	Mozambique	29	14	45	21	42	3	71	43	68	48	45	37	39	9	5
4	Afghanistan	13	2	44	14	105	8	14	2	31	16	25	13	63	11	5
5	Sierra Leone	18	8	31	11	223	10	30	15	56	39	..	..	..	21	12
6	Guinea-Bissau	13	6	50	24	39	..	35	15	76	42	58	32	8	9	4
7	Guinea	21	7	35	13	42	7	27	9	50	24	34	17	44	15	5
8	Malawi	42	18	..	..	238	..	50	26	77	64	55	52	47	6	3
9	Rwanda	43	21	64	37	62	..	65	29	69	68	65	65	36	9	6
10	Mali	11	4	41	24	43	1	13	5	30	17	24	14	40	9	4
11	Liberia	27	8	50	29	225	18	40	13	51x	28x	..	..	..	31x	12x
12	Somalia	5	1	36	14	43	14	6	2	20x	10x	14x	8x	37	12x	7x
13	Chad	20	2	42	18	238	1	29	4	79	35	52	23	71	12	3
14	Eritrea	..	..					..	..							
15	Ethiopia	8	..	33x	16x	191	2	9	3	46	30	32	24	44	17	12
16	Mauritania	..	..	47	21	144	23	12	3	60	42	..	..	68	22	10
17	Zambia	66	37	81	65	77	30	61	40	99	91	81	79	64	25	14
18	Bhutan	..	..	51	25	16	..	5	..	31	20	..	..	26	7	2
19	Nigeria	35	14	62	40	172	32	54	31	82	63	..	..	52	22	17
20	Zaire	61	22	84	61	103	1	89	32	89	67	67	53	73	32	16
21	Uganda	52	30	62	35	101	10	39	18	76	63	57	50	76x	16	8
22	Cambodia	..	23	48	22	113	9	..	..	..	..	..	..	50x	..	..
23	Burundi	29	10	61	40	58	1	33	10	79	64	55	46	83	6	4
24	Central African Rep.	26	6	52	25	66	4	50	11	83	51	66	43	48	17	6
25	Yemen	14	3	53	26	..	..	..	..	111	43	..	..	53	47	10
26	Tanzania, U. Rep. of,	48	18	..	..	24	2	33	16	64	63	46	47	73	5	4
27	Ghana	43	18	70	51	266	15	58	31	82	67	..	..	87	48	31
28	Madagascar	56	43	88	73	200	20	74	57	94	90	64	63	32	20	18
29	Sudan	28	6	43	12	250	71	29	11	58x	41x	..	..	76	23x	17x
30	Gabon	43	22	74	49	141	37	..	..	..	..	..	..	44	..	..
31	Lesotho	49	74	..	..	70	6	73	109	99	115	64	76	50	21	31
32	Burkina Faso	13	3	28	9	26	5	12	5	45	28	36	23	64	9	5
33	Benin	23	8	32	16	90	5	39	15	87	44	69	36	40	16	6
34	Senegal	18	5	52	25	113	36	37	18	67	49	55	41	85	21	11
35	Lao Peo. Dem. Rep.	37	28	92x	76x	126	7	43	20	116	91	..	..	38x	31	21
36	Pakistan	30	11	47	21	87	17	39	11	47	26	..	..	51	29	13
37	Togo	27	7	56	31	211	6	64	25	126	80	85	58	46	33	10
38	Haiti	26x	17x	59	47	46	5	50	39	86	81	44	44	9	20	19
39	Nepal	23	3	38	13	34	2	19	3	112	57	84	43	..	42	17
40	Bangladesh	36	12	47	22	42	5	80	31	78	68	69	61	46	23	12
41	Côte d'Ivoire	26	10	67	40	142	61	62	22	88x	62x	..	..	73	27	12
42	India	47	20	62	34	79	32	83	44	109	83	..	..	53	54	33
43	Bolivia	68	46	85	71	599	163	70	43	87	78	83	75	50	37	31
44	Cameroon	47	19	67	43	139	29	77	37	108	93	80	69	68	31	21
45	Myanmar	85	57	89	72	82	2	60	53	106	100	..	..	..	25	23
46	Indonesia	66	42	88	75	147	60	78	58	119	114	100	96	79	49	41
47	Congo	50	19	70	44	110	6	..	..	..	..	..	..	62	37	14
48	Libyan Arab Jamahiriya	60	13	75	50	224	99	..	..	..	..	..	..	..	..	..
49	Turkmenistan	..	..					..	..							
50	Turkey	69	34	90	71	161	175	90	58	114	105	..	..	97	66	42
51	Zimbabwe	63	47	74	60	85	31	82	65	118	116	..	..	75	54	46
52	Tajikistan	..	..	..	..			..	..							
53	Iraq	50	18	70	49	205	69	94	36	104	87	90	78	58	58	37
54	Mongolia	87	74	..	..	132	41	80	80	96	100	..	..	..	87	96
55	Namibia	..	..	..	..	135	17	..	..	89	99	..	..	..	30	38
56	Papua New Guinea	39	24	65	38	72	2	24	15	77	65	79	67	61	15	10
57	Guatemala	51	37	63	47	65	52	48	39	82	70	..	..	36	20x	17x
58	Nicaragua	58	57	..	..	249	62	57	59	94	101	74	77	29	31	44
59	Kenya	44	19	80	59	125	9	62	29	96	92	92x	89x	62	27	19
60	Algeria	39	11	70	46	233	74	55	37	103	88	94	83	90	66	53
61	South Africa	..	..	78x	75x	326	105	..	..	..	..	..	..	..	..	..
62	Uzbekistan	..	..	..	..			..	..							
63	Brazil	69	63	83	80	379	213	58	56	101x	97x	..	..	22	31x	36x
64	Peru	81	60	91	79	253	97	98	74	125x	120x	..	..	70x	66x	60x
65	El Salvador	61	53	76	70	..	..	59	56	77	·78	69	71	27	26	26
66	Morocco	34	10	61	38	209	74	69	28	81	55	66	45	63	42	30
67	Kyrgyzstan															
68	Philippines	84	81	90	89	138	48	98	93	111	110	100	98	71	72	75
69	Ecuador	75	68	88	84	315	83	82	75	118	117	..	..	63	55	57
70	Botswana	37	44	84	65	115	15	38	43	107	112	88	93	95	44	47
71	Honduras	55	50	75	71	385	72	68	67	108	109	89	94	43x	29x	30x
72	Iran, Islamic Rep. of	40	17	64	43	247	70	59	28	119	106	99	90	91	63	47
73	Egypt	50	20	63	34	324	109	79	52	105	90	..	..	95	92	71
74	Azerbaijan	..	..	..	..			..	..							
75	Dominican Rep.	69	65	85	82	170	84	75	74	95	96	73	73	33	44x	57x

No.	Country	Adult literacy rate 1970		Adult literacy rate 1990		No. of sets per 1000 population 1990		Primary school enrolment ratio 1960 (gross)		Primary school enrolment ratio 1986-91 (gross)		Primary school enrolment ratio 1986-91 (net)		% of grade 1 enrolment reaching final grade of primary school 1988	Secondary school enrolment ratio 1986-91 (gross)	
		male	female	male	female	radio	television	male	female	male	female	male	female		male	female
76	Kazakhstan	..	..	..	..	..	..	..	..	..	..	..	..	..	..	..
77	Viet Nam	..	..	92	84	108	39	103	74	105x	99x	..	..	57x	43x	40x
78	Lebanon	79x	58x	88	73	840	330	112	105	105x	95x	..	..	..	57x	56x
79	China	..	..	84	62	184	31	131	90	140	129	100	100	81	53	41
80	Saudi Arabia	15	2	73	48	318	283	32	3	83	72	69	56	90	55	41
81	Syrian Arab Rep.	60	20	78	51	251	59	89	39	114	102	100	93	85	60	43
82	Tunisia	44	17	74	56	196	80	88	43	122	109	100	91	79	50	40
83	Moldova	..	..	..	..	..	..	..	..	..	..	..	..	..	..	..
84	Albania	..	..	..	..	176	86	102	86	98	98	..	..	91	85	74
85	Armenia	..	..	..	..	..	..	..	..	..	..	..	..	..	..	..
86	Paraguay	85x	75x	92	88	171	59	106	94	109	106	95	94	57	29	31
87	Korea, Dem. Peo. Rep.					119	15	..	..	110	103					
88	Mexico	78	69	90	85	243	139	80	75	113	110	..	..	70	52	53
89	Thailand	86	72	96	90	185	112	97	88	86	85	..	..	59	33	32
90	Russian Federation	..	..	..	..	..	..	..	..	..	..	..	..	..	..	..
91	Oman	..	..	..	..	646	766	..	..	108	99	87	82	91	59	48
92	Jordan	64	29	89	70	254	81	..	..	105x	102x	94x	91x	95	79x	73x
93	Georgia	..	..	..	..	..	..	..	..	..	..	..	..	..	..	..
94	Romania	96	91	..	..	198	194	101	95	86	96	..	..	94	93	90
95	Latvia	..	..	..	..	..	..	..	..	..	..	..	..	..	..	..
96	Ukraine	..	..	..	..	794	327	..	..	..	..	..	..	..	..	..
97	Argentina	94	92	95	95	681	222	99	99	107	114	..	..	..	69	78
98	Estonia	..	..	100x	100x	..	..	..	..	..	..	..	..	..	..	..
99	Mauritius	77	59	..	..	356	215	96	90	102	104	92	94	98	53	53
100	Venezuela	79	71	87	90	436	167	98	99	94	94	60	62	70	30	41
101	Belarus	..	..	..	..	306	268	..	..	..	..	..	..	..	..	..
102	Trinidad and Tobago	95	89	97x	93x	468	302	111	108	95	96	90	90	89	79	82
103	United Arab Emirates	24	7	..	..	324	110	..	..	117	114	100	100	96	63	72
104	Uruguay	93x	93x	97	96	603	233	117	117	107	106	..	..	93	61x	62x
105	Yugoslavia (former)	92	76	97	88	246	198	..	..	95	95	80	79	..	80	79
106	Colombia	79	76	87	86	170	115	74	74	109	111	..	..	56	48	57
107	Lithuania	..	..	99x	98x	..	..	..	..	..	..	..	..	..	..	..
108	Panama	81	81	88	88	223	165	89	86	109	105	91	92	79	57	62
109	Bulgaria	94	89	..	..	438	250	94	92	97	95	85	84	62	72	75
110	Sri Lanka	85	69	93	84	197	35	107	95	108	105	100	100	94	72	77
111	Malaysia	71	48	86	70	429	148	108	79	93	93	..	..	96	55	58
112	Chile	90	88	93	93	342	205	87	86	99	97	..	..	77	71	77
113	Kuwait	65	42	77	67	343	285	132	99	101	99	84	86	90	93	87
114	Poland	98	97	..	..	429	293	110	107	99	98	97	97	92	80	84
115	Hungary	98	98	99x	99x	595	410	103	100	94	94	90	91	94	78	79
116	Costa Rica	88	87	93	93	259	149	94	92	102	101	87	87	77	41	43
117	Jamaica	96	97	98	99	411	130	78	79	104	105	98	100	85	57	63
118	Slovakia	..	..	..	..	..	..	..	..	..	..	..	..	..	..	..
119	Portugal	78	65	89	81	218	177	132	129	121	117	99	100	..	58	59
120	Czech Republic	..	..	..	..	..	..	..	..	..	..	..	..	..	..	..
121	Cuba	86	87	95	93	345	207	109	110	105	100	96	95	88	84	94
122	Israel	93	83	95x	89x	471	266	99	97	92	95	..	..	78	79	86
123	Belgium	99	99	..	..	778	452	111	108	102	103	98	99	78	103	104
124	USA	99	99	..	..	2123	815	..	..	105	104	99	99	90	92	91
125	New Zealand	..	..	..	..	929	442	110	106	106	105	100	100	95	88	91
126	Italy	95	93	98	96	797	424	112	109	96	96	..	..	100	78	78
127	Spain	93	87	97	93	306	396	106	116	109	108	100	100	94	102	112
128	Greece	93	76	98	89	423	196	104	101	100	101	96	97	100	101	97
129	Korea, Rep.	94	81	99	94	1006	210	108	94	106	109	100	100	100	89	86
130	Austria	..	..	..	..	624	481	106	104	103	102	93	93	97	82	85
131	France	99	98	..	..	896	406	144	143	112	110	100	100	96	93	100
132	United Kingdom	..	..	..	..	1146	435	92	92	106	107	100	100	..	82	85
133	Australia	..	..	..	..	1280	486	103	103	105	105	97	97	99	82	85
134	Switzerland	..	..	..	..	155	20	118	118	..	..	..	..	..	..	..
135	Germany	..	..	..	..	..	..	..	..	105	105	89	90	..	99	96
136	Canada	..	..	..	..	1026	641	108	105	106	104	96	97	96	106	107
137	Denmark	..	..	..	..	1030	535	103	103	97	98	..	..	99	108	110
138	Norway	..	..	..	..	798	425	100	100	99	99	99	98	100	98	102
139	Netherlands	..	..	..	..	906	495	105	104	115	118	100	100	94	104	101
140	Sweden	..	..	..	..	888	474	95	96	106	107	100	100	100	89	93
141	Hong Kong	..	..	..	..	649	274	88	72	105	104	95x	95x	98	71	75
142	Singapore	92	55	92x	74x	643	376	120	101	111	109	100	100	100	68	71
143	Finland	..	..	..	..	998	497	100	95	100	99	..	..	100	104	124
144	Japan	99	99	..	..	907	620	103	102	101	101	100	100	100	94	97
145	Ireland	..	..	..	..	583	276	107	112	100	101	87	89	97	93	102

Countries listed in descending order of their 1992 under-five mortality rates (table 1).

Table 5: Demographic indicators

		Population (millions) 1992		Population annual growth rate (%)		Crude death rate		Crude birth rate		Life expectancy		Total fertility rate 1992	% of population urbanized 1992	Average annual growth rate of urban population (%)	
		under 16	under 5	1965-80	1980-92	1960	1992	1960	1992	1960	1992			1965-80	1980-92
1	Niger	4.1	1.7	2.8	3.3	29	19	53	51	35	46	7.1	21	7.2	7.2
2	Angola	4.9	2.0	2.0	2.9	31	19	49	51	33	46	7.2	30	5.5	5.9
3	Mozambique	7.0	2.7	2.5	1.7	26	18	47	45	37	47	6.5	30	9.5	8.7
4	Afghanistan	8.2	3.5	1.9	1.4	30	22	52	52	33	43	6.9	19	5.3	3.1
5	Sierra Leone	2.0	0.8	2.0	2.5	33	22	48	48	32	43	6.5	34	5.1	5.2
6	Guinea-Bissau	0.4	0.2	2.8	2.0	29	22	40	43	34	43	5.8	21	3.9	3.7
7	Guinea	3.0	1.2	1.6	2.6	31	20	53	51	34	44	7.0	27	4.9	5.7
8	Malawi	5.3	2.1	3.0	4.3	28	21	54	55	38	44	7.6	13	7.1	6.9
9	Rwanda	3.9	1.6	3.2	3.1	22	18	50	52	42	46	8.5	6	6.8	4.8
10	Mali	4.8	1.9	2.2	3.0	29	19	52	51	35	46	7.1	25	4.8	5.6
11	Liberia	1.3	0.5	3.0	3.2	25	14	50	47	41	55	6.8	48	6.1	5.8
12	Somalia	4.6	1.8	3.1	2.6	28	19	50	50	36	47	7.0	25	4.0	3.6
13	Chad	2.7	1.0	2.0	2.2	30	18	46	44	35	47	5.9	34	7.5	6.5
14	Eritrea	1.6	0.6	. .	. .	. .	16	. .	42	. .	47	5.8	. .	. .	. .
15	Ethiopia	25.6	10.3	2.4	2.6	28	19	51	49	36	47	7.0	13	4.5	4.3
16	Mauritania	1.0	0.4	2.3	2.7	28	18	48	46	35	48	6.5	50	10.1	7.2
17	Zambia	4.4	1.7	3.1	3.4	22	18	50	47	42	45	6.4	42	6.6	3.9
18	Bhutan	0.7	0.3	1.9	2.2	26	17	42	40	37	48	5.9	6	4.2	5.4
19	Nigeria	57.3	22.1	3.2	3.2	24	14	52	45	40	52	6.5	37	6.3	5.8
20	Zaire	19.9	7.8	2.9	3.3	23	15	47	48	41	52	6.7	29	3.5	3.2
21	Uganda	9.5	3.8	3.3	2.9	21	21	50	51	43	42	7.3	12	5.3	5.4
22	Cambodia	3.8	1.4	0.4	2.5	21	14	45	39	42	51	4.5	12	0.0	3.9
23	Burundi	2.8	1.1	1.7	2.9	23	17	46	46	41	48	6.8	6	6.1	5.2
24	Central African Rep.	1.5	0.6	2.1	2.6	26	18	43	45	39	47	6.2	48	4.5	4.6
25	Yemen	6.5	2.5	2.3	3.5	28	14	53	49	36	52	7.2	31	6.3	7.1
26	Tanzania, U. Rep. of	13.8	5.5	3.0	3.4	23	15	51	48	41	51	6.8	22	9.9	6.9
27	Ghana	7.6	2.9	2.1	3.3	19	12	48	42	45	56	6.0	35	3.3	4.3
28	Madagascar	6.1	2.4	2.5	3.2	24	13	48	45	41	55	6.6	25	5.1	5.9
29	Sudan	12.6	4.7	2.8	3.0	25	14	47	42	39	52	6.1	23	5.6	4.3
30	Gabon	0.4	0.2	3.3	3.6	24	16	31	42	41	53	5.3	48	6.7	6.0
31	Lesotho	0.8	0.3	2.2	2.6	24	10	43	35	43	60	4.7	21	7.1	6.5
32	Burkina Faso	4.4	1.7	2.3	2.6	28	18	49	47	36	48	6.5	17	5.5	8.5
33	Benin	2.4	1.0	2.4	2.9	33	18	47	49	35	46	7.1	40	8.3	4.9
34	Senegal	3.7	1.4	2.8	2.8	27	16	50	43	37	49	6.1	41	3.4	3.9
35	Lao Peo. Dem. Rep.	2.1	0.8	1.8	2.8	23	15	45	45	40	51	6.7	20	5.1	6.1
36	Pakistan	57.3	21.7	2.7	3.2	23	11	49	41	43	59	6.2	33	3.8	4.6
37	Togo	1.8	0.7	3.2	3.0	26	13	48	45	39	55	6.6	30	7.9	5.2
38	Haiti	2.9	1.0	1.7	1.9	23	12	42	35	42	56	4.8	30	3.7	3.9
39	Nepal	9.4	3.4	2.4	2.7	26	13	46	38	38	53	5.5	12	6.6	7.8
40	Bangladesh	51.5	18.2	2.8	2.5	22	14	47	39	40	53	4.8	18	6.7	6.3
41	Côte d'Ivoire	6.6	2.6	4.0	3.8	25	15	53	50	39	52	7.4	42	6.7	5.4
42	India	330.8	112.1	2.2	2.0	21	10	43	29	44	60	3.9	26	3.6	3.1
43	Bolivia	3.2	1.1	2.5	2.5	22	10	46	35	43	61	4.6	52	3.2	3.9
44	Cameroon	5.7	2.1	2.6	2.9	24	12	44	41	39	56	5.7	42	6.9	5.4
45	Myanmar	17.4	6.2	2.2	2.1	21	11	42	33	44	57	4.2	25	3.1	2.6
46	Indonesia	70.5	23.1	2.3	2.0	23	9	44	27	41	62	3.1	30	4.6	4.6
47	Congo	1.1	0.4	2.7	2.9	23	15	45	45	42	52	6.3	42	3.4	4.2
48	Libyan Arab Jamahiriya	2.3	0.9	4.2	3.9	19	8	49	42	47	63	6.4	84	10.4	5.5
49	Turkmenistan	1.7	0.6	. .	. .	. .	8	. .	36	. .	66	4.5	45	. .	. .
50	Turkey	21.6	7.6	2.4	2.3	18	7	45	28	50	67	3.5	64	4.0	5.5
51	Zimbabwe	5.0	1.9	3.1	3.3	20	11	53	41	45	56	5.4	30	6.0	5.8
52	Tajikistan	2.7	1.0	. .	. .	. .	6	. .	41	. .	69	5.3	32	. .	. .
53	Iraq	8.9	3.3	3.3	3.3	20	7	49	39	48	66	5.7	73	5.0	4.2
54	Mongolia	1.0	0.4	2.8	2.7	18	8	43	34	47	63	4.7	59	4.2	3.8
55	Namibia	0.7	0.3	2.7	3.0	22	11	45	43	42	59	6.0	29	4.8	5.1
56	Papua New Guinea	1.7	0.6	2.4	2.3	23	11	44	34	41	56	4.9	17	8.6	4.3
57	Guatemala	4.6	1.7	2.8	2.9	19	8	49	39	46	64	5.4	40	3.4	3.5
58	Nicaragua	2.0	0.7	3.1	2.9	19	7	51	41	47	66	5.1	61	4.6	4.0
59	Kenya	12.8	4.7	3.6	3.5	22	10	53	44	45	59	6.3	25	7.7	7.3
60	Algeria	11.9	3.9	3.0	2.8	20	7	51	34	47	66	4.9	53	4.0	4.6
61	South Africa	16.1	5.5	2.7	2.5	17	9	42	31	49	63	4.1	50	2.8	2.8
62	Uzbekistan	9.4	3.3	. .	. .	. .	6	. .	34	. .	69	2.3	41	. .	. .
63	Brazil	55.2	17.3	2.4	2.0	13	7	43	24	55	66	2.8	77	4.3	3.2
64	Peru	8.8	2.9	2.7	2.2	19	8	47	29	48	64	3.6	71	4.2	3.0
65	El Salvador	2.4	0.8	2.7	1.5	16	7	48	34	50	66	4.1	45	3.2	2.2
66	Morocco	11.1	3.9	2.5	2.6	21	8	50	33	47	63	4.4	47	4.2	3.7
67	Kyrgyzstan	1.8	0.6	. .	. .	. .	8	. .	30	. .	66	3.9	38	. .	. .
68	Philippines	27.0	9.2	2.8	2.4	15	7	45	31	53	65	4.0	44	3.9	3.8
69	Ecuador	4.5	1.5	3.0	2.6	15	7	46	30	53	66	3.7	58	4.6	4.3
70	Botswana	0.6	0.2	3.3	3.1	20	10	52	39	46	61	5.1	28	12.5	8.2
71	Honduras	2.5	0.9	3.1	3.3	19	7	51	37	46	66	5.0	45	5.4	5.3
72	Iran, Islamic Rep. of	29.7	11.1	3.1	3.8	21	7	47	40	50	67	6.0	58	4.9	5.1
73	Egypt	22.5	7.7	2.2	2.5	21	9	45	32	46	61	4.2	44	2.7	2.5
74	Azerbaijan	2.6	0.9	. .	. .	. .	6	. .	26	. .	71	3.2	54	. .	. .
75	Dominican Rep.	2.9	1.0	2.7	2.3	16	6	50	29	52	67	3.4	62	5.1	4.0

		Population (millions) 1992		Population annual growth rate (%)		Crude death rate		Crude birth rate		Life expectancy		Total fertility rate 1992	% of population urbanized 1992	Average annual growth rate of urban population (%)	
		under 16	under 5	1965-80	1980-92	1960	1992	1960	1992	1960	1992			1965-80	1980-92
76	Kazakhstan	5.6	1.9	..	..	..	8	..	21	..	69	2.7	57	..	..
77	Viet Nam	27.9	9.3	2.3	2.2	23	9	41	29	44	64	3.9	20	3.3	2.6
78	Lebanon	1.0	0.4	1.4	0.5	14	7	43	27	60	68	3.1	85	4.1	1.8
79	China	343.8	119.1	2.1	1.5	19	7	37	21	47	71	2.2	28	2.6	4.4
80	Saudi Arabia	7.1	2.6	4.5	4.4	23	5	49	36	44	69	6.4	79	8.1	5.8
81	Syrian Arab Rep.	6.7	2.5	3.3	3.5	18	6	47	43	50	67	6.2	51	4.3	4.3
82	Tunisia	3.3	1.1	2.1	2.3	19	7	47	27	48	68	3.5	57	3.8	3.4
83	Moldova	1.4	0.4	..	..	..	10	..	16	..	68	2.5	47	..	..
84	Albania	1.1	0.4	2.4	1.8	10	5	41	23	62	73	2.7	36	2.9	2.4
85	Armenia	1.1	0.3	..	..	..	7	..	23	..	72	3.0	68	..	..
86	Paraguay	1.9	0.7	2.9	3.0	9	6	43	33	64	67	4.4	49	3.8	4.3
87	Korea, Dem. Peo. Rep.	6.9	2.5	2.6	1.8	13	5	42	24	54	71	2.4	60	4.1	2.3
88	Mexico	34.7	11.6	3.0	2.3	13	6	45	28	57	70	3.2	74	4.2	3.2
89	Thailand	18.5	5.6	2.8	1.5	15	6	44	21	52	69	2.3	24	4.7	4.2
90	Russian Federation	36.1	11.5	..	..	..	12	..	12	..	69	1.8	74	..	..
91	Oman	0.8	0.3	3.7	4.2	28	5	51	41	40	69	6.8	12	7.6	8.0
92	Jordan	2.0	0.7	2.7	3.2	23	6	50	39	47	68	5.7	70	4.4	4.5
93	Georgia	1.4	0.4	..	..	..	9	..	15	..	73	2.1	56	..	..
94	Romania	5.7	1.8	1.0	0.4	9	11	20	16	65	70	2.1	55	2.8	1.3
95	Latvia	0.6	0.2	0.7	0.5	10	12	16	14	70	71	2.0	72	1.6	0.9
96	Ukraine	11.6	3.6	..	..	..	13	..	12	..	70	1.8	67	..	..
97	Argentina	10.3	3.2	1.6	1.3	9	9	24	20	65	71	2.8	87	2.1	1.7
98	Estonia	0.4	0.1	0.9	0.6	11	12	16	14	69	71	2.1	72	1.7	0.8
99	Mauritius	0.3	0.1	1.7	1.1	10	7	44	18	59	70	2.0	41	2.6	0.7
100	Venezuela	7.8	2.5	3.4	2.5	10	5	45	26	60	70	3.2	91	4.6	3.2
101	Belarus	2.5	0.8	..	..	..	11	..	13	..	71	1.9	66	..	..
102	Trinidad and Tobago	0.5	0.1	1.3	1.3	9	6	38	24	63	71	2.8	66	1.2	1.6
103	United Arab Emirates	0.5	0.2	13.0	4.2	19	4	46	21	53	71	4.5	82	15.6	5.3
104	Uruguay	0.8	0.3	0.5	0.6	10	10	22	17	68	72	2.3	89	0.9	1.0
105	Yugoslavia (former)	5.7	1.7	0.9	0.6	10	9	23	14	63	72	1.9	58	3.4	2.6
106	Colombia	12.2	3.8	2.4	1.9	12	6	45	24	57	69	2.7	71	3.6	2.8
107	Lithuania	0.9	0.3	1.0	0.8	8	10	21	15	69	73	2.0	70	3.0	1.9
108	Panama	0.9	0.3	2.6	2.1	10	5	41	25	61	73	2.9	54	3.3	2.7
109	Bulgaria	1.9	0.6	0.5	0.1	9	12	18	13	68	72	1.8	69	2.4	1.1
110	Sri Lanka	6.0	1.8	1.9	1.5	9	6	36	21	62	71	2.5	22	2.4	1.6
111	Malaysia	7.5	2.6	2.5	2.6	15	5	44	29	54	71	3.7	45	4.4	4.7
112	Chile	4.4	1.5	1.7	1.7	13	6	37	23	57	72	2.7	85	2.6	2.1
113	Kuwait	0.8	0.3	7.1	3.0	10	2	44	28	60	75	3.7	96	8.1	3.4
114	Poland	10.1	2.9	0.8	0.6	8	10	24	14	67	72	2.1	63	1.8	1.3
115	Hungary	2.2	0.6	0.4	-0.2	10	14	16	12	68	70	1.8	66	1.9	1.0
116	Costa Rica	1.2	0.4	2.9	2.8	10	4	47	27	62	76	3.2	48	3.7	3.7
117	Jamaica	0.8	0.3	1.3	1.2	9	6	39	22	63	73	2.4	54	2.7	2.4
118	Slovakia	1.4	0.4	..	..	..	10	..	15	..	72	2.0	..	..	..
119	Portugal	2.1	0.6	0.5	0.1	11	10	24	12	63	75	1.5	35	1.8	1.5
120	Czech Republic	2.3	0.7	..	..	..	11	..	13	..	72	1.9	..	..	..
121	Cuba	2.6	0.9	1.5	0.9	9	7	31	17	64	76	1.9	75	2.6	1.7
122	Israel	1.6	0.5	2.8	2.3	6	7	27	21	69	76	2.9	92	3.4	2.7
123	Belgium	1.9	0.6	0.3	0.1	12	11	17	12	70	76	1.6	96	0.4	0.2
124	USA	58.8	19.2	1.1	1.0	9	9	23	16	70	76	2.1	76	1.2	1.2
125	New Zealand	0.8	0.3	1.1	0.9	9	8	26	17	71	76	2.1	84	1.5	0.9
126	Italy	10.3	2.9	0.5	0.2	10	10	18	10	69	77	1.3	70	1.0	0.6
127	Spain	7.9	2.1	1.1	0.3	9	9	21	11	69	77	1.4	79	2.2	1.1
128	Greece	2.0	0.5	0.8	0.5	8	10	19	10	69	77	1.5	63	2.1	1.3
129	Korea, Rep. of	11.7	3.4	1.9	1.2	14	6	43	16	54	71	1.8	74	5.7	3.5
130	Austria	1.4	0.4	0.3	0.3	12	11	18	12	69	76	1.5	59	0.8	0.9
131	France	12.3	3.8	0.7	0.5	12	10	18	14	70	77	1.8	73	1.3	0.4
132	United Kingdom	11.8	3.9	0.2	0.2	12	11	17	14	71	76	1.9	89	0.4	0.2
133	Australia	4.1	1.3	1.7	1.5	9	8	22	15	71	77	1.9	85	1.9	1.4
134	Switzerland	1.2	0.4	0.5	0.6	10	10	18	13	71	78	1.6	63	1.0	1.4
135	Germany	14.5	4.6	0.2	0.2	12	11	17	11	70	76	1.5	86	0.6	0.5
136	Canada	6.1	1.9	1.3	1.1	8	8	26	14	71	77	1.8	78	1.6	1.3
137	Denmark	0.9	0.3	0.5	0.1	9	12	17	12	72	76	1.7	85	1.0	0.2
138	Norway	0.9	0.3	0.6	0.4	9	11	18	15	73	77	2.0	76	2.0	1.0
139	Netherlands	3.0	1.0	0.9	0.6	8	9	21	14	73	77	1.7	89	1.2	0.6
140	Sweden	1.7	0.6	0.5	0.3	10	11	15	14	73	78	2.1	84	1.0	0.5
141	Hong Kong	1.3	0.4	2.1	1.2	7	6	35	13	66	78	1.4	95	2.5	1.4
142	Singapore	0.7	0.2	1.7	1.1	8	6	38	16	64	74	1.7	100	1.7	1.1
143	Finland	1.0	0.3	0.3	0.4	9	10	19	13	68	76	1.8	60	2.4	0.4
144	Japan	23.7	6.8	1.1	0.5	8	7	18	11	68	79	1.7	77	1.9	0.7
145	Ireland	1.0	0.3	1.1	0.2	12	9	21	15	70	75	2.1	58	2.0	0.5

Countries listed in descending order of their 1992 under-five mortality rates (table 1).

Table 6: Economic indicators

		GNP per capita (US$) 1991	GNP per capita average annual growth rate (%)		Rate of inflation (%) 1980-91	% of population below absolute poverty level 1980-89		% of central government expenditure allocated to (1986-92)			ODA inflow in millions US$ 1991	ODA inflow as a % of recipient GNP 1991	Debt service as a % of exports of goods and services	
			1965-80	1980-91		urban	rural	health	education	defence			1970	1991
1	Niger	300	-2.5	-4.1	2	. .	35x	. .	. .	. .	418	18	4	30
2	Angola	610x	. .	6.1x		. .	. .	6x	15x	34x	250	. .	. .	4
3	Mozambique	80		-1.1	38	50	67	5	10	35x	1022	79	. .	11
4	Afghanistan	280x	0.6		. .	18x	36x	. .	. .	. .	521		. .	. .
5	Sierra Leone	210	0.7	-1.6	59	. .	65x	10	13	10	108	12	11	4x
6	Guinea-Bissau	180	-2.7	1.1	56	. .	. .	1	3	4	123	68	. .	26x
7	Guinea	460	1.3		. .	. .	. .		11x	29x	331	12		14
8	Malawi	230	3.2	0.1	15	25	85	7	9	5	494	24	8	16x
9	Rwanda	270	1.6	-2.4	4	30	90x	5x	26x	. .	328	17	1	14
10	Mali	280	2.1x	-0.1	4	27x	48x	2	9	8	408	17	1	3
11	Liberia	450x	0.5	5.2x	. .	. .	23x	5	11	9	143	. .	8	. .
12	Somalia	150x	-0.1	-1.8x	50x	40x	70x	1x	2x	38x	282	. .	2	8x
13	Chad	210	-1.9	3.8	1	30x	56x	8x	8x	. .	269	22	4	4
14	Eritrea	120												
15	Ethiopia	120	0.4	-1.6	2	60	65	3	11	. .	951	15	11	23
16	Mauritania	510	-0.1	-1.8	9	. .	. .	4x	23x	. .	208	20	3	12
17	Zambia	420x	-1.2	-2.9x	42x	25		7	9	. .	587	. .	6	12x
18	Bhutan	180		6.8	8	. .	. .	5	11	. .	55	21	. .	7x
19	Nigeria	340	4.2	-2.3	18	. .	. .	1	3	3	293	1	4	25
20	Zaire	230x	-1.3	-1.6	61x	. .	80x	4x	6x	14x	505	. .	4	6x
21	Uganda	170	-2.2	3.3	107x	. .	. .	2x	15x	26x	566	20	3	42
22	Cambodia	200x			. .	. .	. .	. .	. .	. .	62	4	. .	. .
23	Burundi	210	2.4	1.3	4	55x	85x	4x	16x	16x	249	21	2	30
24	Central African Rep.	390	0.8	-1.4	5	. .	91	. .	. .	. .	225	19	5	5
25	Yemen	520	. .	. .	. .	. .	. .	5	21	21	. .	. .	. .	8
26	Tanzania, U. Rep. of	100	0.8	-0.8	26	. .	. .	6x	8x	16x	1038	41	5	19x
27	Ghana	400	-0.8	-0.3	40	59	37	9	26	3	603	10	6	15
28	Madagascar	210	-0.4	-2.5	17	50x	50x	7	17	8	358	14	4	24
29	Sudan	420x	0.8	-2.4	34x	. .	85x	. .	. .	. .	836	. .	11	4
30	Gabon	3780	5.6	-4.2	2	. .	. .	. .	. .	. .	142	3	6	6x
31	Lesotho	580	6.8	-0.5	14	50x	55x	11	22	6	125	12	5	5
32	Burkina Faso	290	1.7	1.2	4	. .	. .	5	14	18	379	14	7	8x
33	Benin	380	-0.3	-0.9	2	. .	. .	6x	31x	17x	270	15	2	7
34	Senegal	720	-0.5	0.1	6	. .	. .	. .	. .	. .	769	14	3	14x
35	Lao Peo. Dem. Rep.	220	. .	1.2	. .	. .	. .	. .	. .	. .	161	17	. .	8x
36	Pakistan	400	1.8	3.2	7	32x	29x	1	2x	28x	1183	3	24	22x
37	Togo	410	1.7	-1.3	4	42x	. .	5	20	11	201	13	3	5
38	Haiti	370	0.9	-2.4	7	65	80	. .	. .	. .	197	8	59	5
39	Nepal	180	. .	2.1	9	55x	61x	5	11	6	403	12	3	12
40	Bangladesh	220	-0.3	1.9	9	86x	86x	5x	11x	10x	2142	9	. .	19
41	Côte d'Ivoire	690	2.8	-4.6	4	30	26	4x	. .	. .	597	7	7	14
42	India	330	1.5	3.2	8	29	33	2	2	17	1657	1	22	27
43	Bolivia	650	1.7	-2.0	263	. .	. .	3	19	13	540	11	11	24
44	Cameroon	850	2.4	-1.0	5	15x	40x	3	12	7	507	5	3	13x
45	Myanmar	220x	1.6	. .	. .	40x	40x	7	16	22	167	. .	12	. .
46	Indonesia	610	5.2	3.9	9	20	16	2	9	8	1733	2	7	21
47	Congo	1120	2.7	-0.2	0	. .	. .	. .	. .	. .	134	5	12	19
48	Libyan Arab Jamahiriya	5310x	0.0	-9.2x	0x	. .	. .	. .	. .	. .	19	. .	. .	. .
49	Turkmenistan	1700		0.7	. .	. .	. .	. .	. .	. .	. .	. .	. .	. .
50	Turkey	1780	3.6	2.9	45	. .	. .	3	18	10	1640	2	22	29
51	Zimbabwe	650	1.7	-0.2	13	. .	. .	8x	. .	17x	376	6	2	23
52	Tajikistan	1050	. .	-0.1	. .	. .	. .	. .	. .	. .	. .	. .	. .	. .
53	Iraq	1500x	. .	. .	. .	. .	. .	. .	. .	. .	417	. .	. .	. .
54	Mongolia	780x	. .	. .	-1x	. .	. .	. .	. .	. .	18	. .	. .	. .
55	Namibia	1460	. .	-1.2	13	. .	. .	10	22	7	179	8	. .	. .
56	Papua New Guinea	830	. .	-0.6	5	10x	75x	9	15	5	381	12	1	14
57	Guatemala	930	3.0	-1.8	16	17	51	10	20	13	189	2	7	15
58	Nicaragua	460	-0.7	-4.4	584	21x	19x	11x	9x	50x	680	39	11	111
59	Kenya	340	3.1	0.3	9	10x	55x	5	20	10	884	10	6	22x
60	Algeria	1980	4.2	-0.7	10	20x	. .	. .	. .	. .	351	1	4	69
61	South Africa	2560	3.2	0.7	14	. .	. .	. .	. .	. .	. .	. .	. .	. .
62	Uzbekistan	1350	. .	0.8	. .	. .	. .	. .	. .	. .	. .	. .	. .	. .
63	Brazil	2940	6.3	0.5	328	9	34	7	3	4	196	0	13	22
64	Peru	1070	0.8	-2.4	287	46	83	6	21	18	339	1	12	18
65	El Salvador	1080	1.5	-0.3	17	20	32	8	14	21	. .	. .	4	. .
66	Morocco	1030	2.7	1.6	7	28x	45x	3	17	15	1203	5	9	32
67	Kyrgyzstan	1550	. .	2.1	. .	. .	. .	. .	. .	. .	4	0	. .	. .
68	Philippines	730	3.2	-1.2	15	52	64	4	16	11	1231	3	8	19
69	Ecuador	1000	5.4	-0.6	38	40	65	11	18	13	208	2	9	27
70	Botswana	2530	9.9	5.6	13	40	55	5	21	13	131	4	1	3
71	Honduras	580	1.1	-0.5	7	31	70	. .	. .	7x	332	11	3	25
72	Iran, Islamic Rep. of	2170	2.9	-1.3	14	. .	. .	8	21	10	81	0	. .	1
73	Egypt	610	2.8	1.9	13	34	34	3	13	13	4638	14	38	17
74	Azerbaijan	1670	. .	0.4	. .	. .	. .	. .	. .	. .	. .	. .	. .	. .
75	Dominican Rep.	940	3.8	-0.2	25	45x	43x	14	10	5	95	1	4	9

		GNP per capita (US$) 1991	GNP per capita average annual growth rate (%)		Rate of inflation (%) 1980-91	% of population below absolute poverty level 1980-89		% of central government expenditure allocated to (1986-92)			ODA inflow in millions US$ 1991	ODA inflow as a % of recipient GNP 1991	Debt service as a % of exports of goods and services	
			1965-80	1980-91		urban	rural	health	education	defence			1970	1991
76	Kazakhstan	2470	..	0.9	..	..	..	..	..	..	..	..	..	..
77	Viet Nam	240x	..	..	..	..	..	..	..	..	218	..	..	..
78	Lebanon	2150x	..	..	..	..	..	..	..	..	138	..	..	..
79	China	370	4.1	7.8	6	..	13	..	..	8x	2166	1	..	10
80	Saudi Arabia	7820	4.0x	-3.4	-2	..	..	..	..	..	43	0	..	..
81	Syrian Arab Rep.	1160	5.1	-1.4	14	..	..	2	7	32	219	2	11	27x
82	Tunisia	1500	4.7	1.1	7	20x	15x	6	17	6	312	3	20	21
83	Moldova	2170	..	1.8	..	..	..	..	..	..	..	..	..	..
84	Albania	790x	..	..	..	..	..	..	..	..	303	..	..	..
85	Armenia	2150	..	2.1	..	..	..	..	..	..	..	..	..	..
86	Paraguay	1270	4.1	-0.8	25	19x	50x	4	13	13	111	2	12	16x
87	Korea, Dem. Peo. Rep.	970x	..	..	..	..	..	..	..	..	8	..	..	..
88	Mexico	3030	3.6	-0.5	67	..	..	2	14	2	183	0	24	22
89	Thailand	1570	4.4	5.9	4	10	25	7	20	17	738	1	3	5
90	Russian Federation	3220	..	1.3	..	..	..	..	..	..	..	..	..	..
91	Oman	6120	9.0	4.4	-3	..	..	5	11	35	15	0	..	13x
92	Jordan	1050	5.8x	-1.7	2	14x	17x	5	15	21	668	17	4	22
93	Georgia	1640	..	2.2	..	..	..	..	..	..	..	..	..	..
94	Romania	1390	..	0.0	6	..	..	9	10	10	..	..	..	1
95	Latvia	3410	..	2.8	..	..	..	..	..	..	..	..	..	..
96	Ukraine	2340	..	2.3	..	..	..	..	..	..	..	..	..	..
97	Argentina	2790	1.7	-1.5	417	..	..	3	10	10	255	0	22	37
98	Estonia	3830	..	2.1	..	..	..	..	..	..	..	..	..	..
99	Mauritius	2410	3.7	6.1	8	12x	12x	9	15	2	95	4	3	6
100	Venezuela	2730x	2.3	-1.3	21	..	..	10	20	6x	81	0	..	13
101	Belarus	3110	..	3.3	..	..	..	..	..	..	..	..	..	..
102	Trinidad and Tobago	3670	3.1	-5.2	7	..	39x	..	..	..	9	0	5	15x
103	United Arab Emirates	19860x	..	-5.8	1x	..	..	7	15	44	6	0	..	..
104	Uruguay	2840	2.5	-0.4	64	22	..	4	7	9	59	1	22	27
105	Yugoslavia (former)	3060x	5.2	-1.4	123	..	..	..	..	53	130	..	10	14
106	Colombia	1260	3.7	1.2	25	32	70	..	..	..	143	0	12	32
107	Lithuania	2710	..	2.5	..	..	..	..	..	..	..	..	..	..
108	Panama	2130	2.8	-1.8	2	21x	30x	21	17	5	112	2	8	3
109	Bulgaria	1840	..	1.7	8	..	..	5	6	6	..	..	..	21
110	Sri Lanka	500	2.8	2.5	11	..	..	5	8	9	651	8	11	11
111	Malaysia	2520	4.7	2.9	2	13	38	5	19	12	459	1	4	7
112	Chile	2160	0.0	1.6	21	12	20	6	10	8	122	0	19	24
113	Kuwait	16150x	0.6x	-2.2x	-3x	..	..	7	14	20	..	..	..	..
114	Poland	1790	..	0.6	63	..	..	..	..	..	..	..	..	5
115	Hungary	2720	5.1	0.7	10	..	..	8x	3x	4x	..	..	..	30
116	Costa Rica	1850	3.3	0.7	23	8	20	32	19	2	193	3	10	15
117	Jamaica	1380	-0.1	0.0	20	..	80	7x	11x	8x	197	6	3	24
118	Slovakia	..	..	..	..	..	..	..	..	..	..	..	..	..
119	Portugal	5930	4.6	3.1	17	..	..	..	..	6x	..	..	7	22
120	Czech Republic	..	..	..	..	..	..	..	..	..	..	..	..	..
121	Cuba	1170x	..	..	..	..	..	23x	10x	..	42	..	..	..
122	Israel	11950	3.7	1.7	89	..	..	4	10	22	1365	2	3	..
123	Belgium	18950	3.6	2.0	4	..	..	12x	2x	5x	..	..	..	..
124	USA	22240	1.8	1.7	4	..	..	14	2	22	..	..	..	..
125	New Zealand	12350	1.7	0.7	10	..	..	12	12	4	..	..	..	..
126	Italy	18520	3.2	2.2	10	..	..	11x	8x	4x	..	..	..	..
127	Spain	12450	4.1	2.8	9	..	..	14	6	5	..	..	..	..
128	Greece	6340	4.8	1.1	18	..	..	..	..	..	36	0	9	..
129	Korea, Rep. of	6330	7.3	8.7	6	18x	11x	1	16	22	64	0	20	6x
130	Austria	20140	4.0	2.1	4	..	..	13	9	2	..	..	..	..
131	France	20380	3.7	1.8	6	..	..	15x	7x	7x	..	..	..	..
132	United Kingdom	16550	2.0	2.6	6	..	..	13	3	11	..	..	..	..
133	Australia	17050	2.2	1.6	7	..	..	13	7	9	..	..	..	..
134	Switzerland	33610	1.5	1.6	4	..	..	13	3	10	..	..	..	..
135	Germany	23650	3.0x	2.2	3	..	..	19x	1x	8x	..	..	..	..
136	Canada	20440	3.3	2.0	4	..	..	5	3	7	..	..	..	..
137	Denmark	23700	2.2	2.2	5	..	..	1x	9x	5x	..	..	..	..
138	Norway	24220	3.6	2.3	5	..	..	10	9	8	..	..	..	..
139	Netherlands	18780	2.7	1.6	2	..	..	12	11	5	..	..	..	..
140	Sweden	25110	2.0	1.7	7	..	..	1	9	6	..	..	..	..
141	Hong Kong	13430	6.2	5.6	8	..	..	..	17x	..	34	0	..	..
142	Singapore	14210	8.3	5.3	2	..	..	5	20	24	-18	..	1	..
143	Finland	23980	3.6	2.5	7	..	..	11	15	5	..	..	..	..
144	Japan	26930	5.1	3.6	2	..	..	..	..	..	..	..	..	..
145	Ireland	11120	2.8	3.3	6	..	..	13	12	3	..	..	..	..

Countries listed in descending order of their 1992 under-five mortality rates (table 1).

Table 7: Women

		Life expectancy females as a % of males 1992	Adult literacy rate females as a % of males 1990	Enrolment ratios females as a % of males 1986-91		Contraceptive prevalence (%) 1980-93	Pregnant women immunized against tetanus 1990-92	% of births attended by trained health personnel 1983-92	Maternal mortality rate 1980-91
				primary school	secondary school				
1	Niger	107	43	57	44	4	45	15	700
2	Angola	107	52	93	. .	1x	8	15	. .
3	Mozambique	107	47	71	56	4	32	25	300
4	Afghanistan	102	32	52	45	2x	9	9	640
5	Sierra Leone	108	35	70	57	4	80	25	450
6	Guinea-Bissau	108	48	55	44	1x	35	27	700x
7	Guinea	102	37	48	33	1x	70	25	800
8	Malawi	103	. .	83	50	13	66	55	400
9	Rwanda	107	58	99	67	21	88	29	210
10	Mali	107	59	57	44	5	8	32	2000
11	Liberia	105	58	55x	39x	6	20	58	. .
12	Somalia	107	39	50x	58x	1	5x	2	1100
13	Chad	107	43	44	25	1x	5	15	960
14	Eritrea	. .	. .	. .	. .	. .	. .	. .	. .
15	Ethiopia	107	48x	65	71	2	7	14	560x
16	Mauritania	107	45	70	45	4	40	40	. .
17	Zambia	103	80	92	56	15	20	51	150
18	Bhutan	103	49	65	29	2	43	7	1310
19	Nigeria	107	65	77	77	6	25	37	800
20	Zaire	106	73	75	50	1x	29x	. .	800
21	Uganda	105	56	83	50	5	16	38	300
22	Cambodia	106	46	. .	. .		22	47	500
23	Burundi	107	66	81	67	9	56	19	. .
24	Central African Rep.	110	48	61	35	. .	87	66	600
25	Yemen	101	49	39	21	7	13	16	. .
26	Tanzania, U. Rep. of	106	. .	98	80	10	15	53	340x
27	Ghana	107	73	82	65	13	9	40	1000
28	Madagascar	106	83	96	90	17	2	58	570
29	Sudan	105	28	71x	74x	9	14	69	550
30	Gabon	106	66	. .	. .	. .	86	80	190
31	Lesotho	109	. .	116	148	5x	40	40	. .
32	Burkina Faso	107	32	62	56	8	26	42	810
33	Benin	107	50	51	38	9	83	45	160
34	Senegal	104	48	73	52	11	26	41	600
35	Lao Peo. Dem. Rep.	106	83x	78	68	. .	19	. .	300
36	Pakistan	100	45	55	45	12	42	35	500
37	Togo	107	55	63	30	34	81	54	420
38	Haiti	106	80	94	95	10	5	20	340
39	Nepal	98	34	51	40	14	18	6	830
40	Bangladesh	99	47	87	52	31	80	5	600
41	Côte d'Ivoire	106	60	70	44	3	35	50	. .
42	India	101	55	76	61	43	77	33	460
43	Bolivia	108	84	90	84	30	52	55	600
44	Cameroon	106	64	86	68	13	7	64	430
45	Myanmar	106	81	94	92	13	72	57	460
46	Indonesia	106	85	96	84	48	60	32	450
47	Congo	110	63	. .	38x	. .	60	. .	900
48	Libyan Arab Jamahiriya	106	67	. .	. .	. .	16	76	70x
49	Turkmenistan	. .	. .	. .	. .	. .	. .	. .	. .
50	Turkey	108	79	92	64	63	22	77	150
51	Zimbabwe	105	81	98	85	43	60	70	. .
52	Tajikistan	. .	. .	. .	. .	. .	. .	. .	. .
53	Iraq	105	70	84	64	18	45	50	120
54	Mongolia	104	. .	104	110	. .	. .	99	140
55	Namibia	104	. .	111	127	26	52	68	370x
56	Papua New Guinea	103	58	84	67	4	52	20	900
57	Guatemala	108	75	85	85x	23	18	51	200
58	Nicaragua	106	. .	107	142	27	12	73	. .
59	Kenya	107	74	96	70	27	37	50	170x
60	Algeria	104	66	85	80	51	27	15	140x
61	South Africa	110	96x	. .	. .	48	. .	. .	84x
62	Uzbekistan	. .	. .	. .	. .	. .	. .	. .	. .
63	Brazil	109	96	96x	116x	66	21	95	200
64	Peru	106	87	96x	91x	59	27	52	300
65	El Salvador	108	92	101	100	47	26	66	. .
66	Morocco	106	62	68	71	42	80	26	300x
67	Kyrgyzstan	. .	. .	. .	. .	. .	. .	. .	. .
68	Philippines	106	99	99	104	36	52	55	100
69	Ecuador	107	95	99	104	53	5	84	170
70	Botswana	110	77	105	107	33	46	78	250
71	Honduras	107	95	101	103x	41	16	81	220
72	Iran, Islamic Rep. of	102	67	89	75	23x	87	70	120
73	Egypt	104	54	86	77	47	70	41	270
74	Azerbaijan	. .	. .	. .	. .	. .	. .	. .	. .
75	Dominican Rep.	107	96	101	130x	56	24	92	. .

		Life expectancy females as a % of males 1992	Adult literacy rate females as a % of males 1990	Enrolment ratios females as a % of males 1986-91		Contraceptive prevalence (%) 1980-93	Pregnant women immunized against tetanus 1990-92	% of births attended by trained health personnel 1983-92	Maternal mortality rate 1980-91
				primary school	secondary school				
76	Kazakhstan	. .	. .	. .	. .	. .	. .	. .	. .
77	Viet Nam	107	91	94x	93x	53	42	95	120
78	Lebanon	106	83	90x	98x	55x	. .	45	
79	China	105	74	92	77	83	3	94	95
80	Saudi Arabia	104	66	87	75	. .	62	90	41
81	Syrian Arab Rep.	106	65	89	72	52	63	61	140
82	Tunisia	103	76	89	80	50	44	69	70
83	Moldova	. .	. .	. .	. .	. .	. .	. .	. .
84	Albania	109	. .	100	87	. .	. .	99	. .
85	Armenia	. .	. .	. .	. .	. .	. .	. .	. .
86	Paraguay	107	96	97	107	48	54	66	300
87	Korea, Dem. Peo. Rep.	109	. .	94	. .	. .	97	100	41
88	Mexico	110	94	97	102	53	42	77	110
89	Thailand	108	94	99	97	66	72	71	50
90	Russian Federation	. .	. .	. .	. .	. .	. .	. .	. .
91	Oman	106	. .	92	81	9	97	60	. .
92	Jordan	106	79	97x	92x	35	32	87	48x
93	Georgia	. .	. .	. .	. .	. .	. .	. .	. .
94	Romania	109	. .	112	97	58x	. .	100	72
95	Latvia	114	. .	. .	. .	. .	. .	. .	. .
96	Ukraine	. .	. .	. .	. .	. .	. .	. .	. .
97	Argentina	110	100	107	113	74	. .	87	140
98	Estonia	114	100x	. .	. .	. .	. .	. .	. .
99	Mauritius	110	89x	102	100	75	77	85	99
100	Venezuela	109	103	100	137	49x	. .	69	. .
101	Belarus	. .	. .	. .	. .	. .	. .	. .	. .
102	Trinidad and Tobago	107	96x	101	104	53	. .	98	110
103	United Arab Emirates	106	66x	97	114	. .	. .	99	. .
104	Uruguay	109	99	99	102x	. .	13	96	36
105	Yugoslavia (former)	109	91	100	99	55x	. .	86	27
106	Colombia	109	99	102	119	66	40	94	200
107	Lithuania	113	99	. .	. .	. .	. .	. .	. .
108	Panama	106	100	96	109	58	27	96	60
109	Bulgaria	109	. .	98	104	76x	. .	100	9
110	Sri Lanka	106	90	97	107	62	67	94	80
111	Malaysia	106	81	100	105	51	83	87	59
112	Chile	110	100	98	108	43x	. .	98	67
113	Kuwait	106	87	98	94	. .	22	99	6
114	Poland	113	. .	99	105	75x	. .	100	11
115	Hungary	112	100x	100	101	73	. .	99	15
116	Costa Rica	106	100	99	105	70	68	93	36
117	Jamaica	106	101	101	111	55	50	82	120
118	Slovakia	. .	. .	. .	. .	. .	. .	. .	. .
119	Portugal	110	91	97	102	66x	. .	90	10
120	Czech Republic	. .	. .	. .	. .	. .	. .	. .	. .
121	Cuba	105	98	95	112	70	98	90	39
122	Israel	105	94x	103	109	. .	. .	99	3
123	Belgium	109	. .	101	101	81	. .	100	3
124	USA	109	. .	99	99	74	. .	99	8
125	New Zealand	108	. .	99	103	70x	. .	99	13
126	Italy	109	98	100	100	78x	. .	. .	4
127	Spain	108	96	99	110	59	. .	96	5
128	Greece	107	91	101	96	. .	. .	97	5
129	Korea, Rep. of	109	95	103	97	77	. .	89	26
130	Austria	109	. .	99	104	71	. .	. .	8
131	France	111	. .	98	108	79x	. .	94	9
132	United Kingdom	107	. .	101	104	72	. .	100	8
133	Australia	109	. .	100	104	67x	. .	99	3
134	Switzerland	109	. .	. .	. .	71	. .	99	5
135	Germany	109	. .	100	97	. .	. .	99	5
136	Canada	109	. .	98	101	73	. .	99	5
137	Denmark	108	. .	101	102	63x	. .	100	3
138	Norway	109	. .	100	104	71x	. .	. .	3
139	Netherlands	108	. .	103	97	76	. .	100	10
140	Sweden	108	. .	101	104	78	. .	100	5
141	Hong Kong	107	. .	99	106	81	. .	100	6
142	Singapore	108	80x	98	104	74	. .	100	10
143	Finland	111	. .	99	119	80x	. .	100	11
144	Japan	108	. .	100	103	64	. .	100	11
145	Ireland	108	. .	101	110	. .	. .	. .	2

Countries listed in descending order of their under-five mortality rates (table 1).

Table 8: Basic indicators on less populous countries

		Under-5 mortality rate		Infant mortality rate (under 1)		Total population (thousands)	Annual no. of births (thousands)	Annual no. of under-5 deaths (thousands)	GNP per capita (US$)	Life expectancy at birth (years)	Total adult literacy rate	% of age-group enrolled in primary school (gross)	% of children immunized against measles
		1960	1992	1960	1992	1992	1992	1992	1991	1992	1985-90	1986-91	1991-92
1	Gambia	375	220	213	133	908	40.3	8.8	360	45	27	64	83
2	Equatorial Guinea	316	182	188	118	369	16.2	3.0	330	48	50x	134x	66
3	Djibouti	289	158	186	113	467	21.9	3.5	1210	49	12	47	83
4	Comoros	248	130	165	90	585	28.7	3.7	500	56	48x	75	32
5	Swaziland	233	107	157	74	792	29.6	3.2	1050	58	67	104	85
6	Marshall Islands	..	92	..	63	49	1.4	0.1	*	..	91	95	86
7	Sao Tome and Principe	..	85	..	65	124	4.5	0.4	400	68	57x	..	61
8	Vanuatu	..	85	..	65	157	6.0	0.5	1150	65	64	103	74
9	Kiribati	..	81	..	60	74	2.4	0.2	720	56	93	91	77
10	Maldives	258	78	158	56	227	8.8	0.7	460	63	91	87	98
11	Guyana	126	65	100	49	808	20.7	1.3	430	65	96x	115	76
12	Cape Verde	164	60	110	44	384	13.8	0.8	750	68	37x	116	82
13	Samoa	..	58	..	45	158	5.2	0.3	960	66	98	100	91
14	Tuvalu	..	56	..	40	12	..	0.0	650	..	99	101	63
15	Belize	..	52	..	41	198	7.2	0.4	2010	69	93	90	72
16	Saint Kitts and Nevis	..	42	..	34	42	0.8	0.0	3960	71	90	..	99
17	Suriname	96	35	70	28	438	11.4	0.4	3630	70	95	132	84
18	Grenada	..	35	..	29	91	2.2	0.1	2180	71	96x	88x	73
19	Palau	..	35	..	25	16	0.5	0.0	790	..	98	103	94
20	Solomon Islands	185	34	120	27	342	12.9	0.4	560	70	62	93	74
21	Qatar	239	33	145	27	453	10.4	0.3	14770	70	76	97	79
22	British Virgin Islands	..	33x	..	27x	17	0.3	0.0x	8500	75	98x	..	99
23	Turks and Caicos Islands	..	31x	..	25x	13	0.2	0.0x	780	..	98x	..	59
24	Bahamas	68	29	51	24	264	5.2	0.2	11750	72	..	..	93
25	Fiji	97	29	71	24	739	17.6	0.5	1930	71	87	123	91
26	Micronesia, Fed. States of	..	29	..	25	109	3.7	0.4	*	71	81	100	88
27	Cook Islands	..	28	..	26	17	0.4	0.0	1550	..	99	98	87
28	Antigua and Barbuda	..	25	..	20	66	1.1	0.0	4430	74	95	100	87
29	Saint Vincent / Grenadines	..	25	..	20	109	2.4	0.1	1730	71	82	95x	100
30	Tonga	..	25	..	21	97	2.9	0.1	1280	68	99	98	90
31	Dominica	..	22	..	18	72	1.5	0.0	2440	73	94x	..	98
32	Saint Lucia	..	21	..	17	137	3.8	0.1	2490	72	82x	95x	97
33	Seychelles	..	20	..	16	72	1.6	0.0	5110	71	88	102x	92
34	Bahrain	208	16	130	13	533	14.1	0.2	7130	71	77x	103	87
35	Montserrat	..	15	..	12	11	0.2	0.0	3330	75	97x	100x	100
36	Barbados	90	12	74	10	259	4.1	0.0	6630	76	98	114	90
37	Malta	42	11	37	9	359	5.5	0.1	7280	76	86	109	80
38	Cyprus	36	11	30	9	716	12.3	0.1	8640	77	94	103	74
39	Luxembourg	41	11	33	9	378	4.7	0.1	31780	75	..	93	80
40	Brunei Darussalam	87	10	63	8	270	6.5	0.1	20760	74	78x	..	99
41	Iceland	22	7	17	6	260	4.5	0.0	23170	78	..	101	99

* Range $1500 - $3499.

MEASURING HUMAN DEVELOPMENT
An introduction to table 9

If development in the 1990s is to assume a more human face then there arises a corresponding need for a means of measuring human as well as economic progress. From UNICEF's point of view, in particular, there is a need for an agreed method of measuring the level of child well-being and its rate of change.

The under-five mortality rate (U5MR) is used in table 9 (next page) as the principal indicator of such progress.

The U5MR has several advantages. First, it measures an end result of the development process rather than an 'input' such as school enrolment level, per capita calorie availability, or the number of doctors per thousand population – all of which are means to an end.

Second, the U5MR is known to be the result of a wide variety of inputs: the nutritional health and the health knowledge of mothers; the level of immunization and ORT use; the availability of maternal and child health services (including prenatal care); income and food availability in the family; the availability of clean water and safe sanitation; and the overall safety of the child's environment.

Third, the U5MR is less susceptible than, say, per capita GNP to the fallacy of the average. This is because the natural scale does not allow the children of the rich to be one thousand times as likely to survive, even if the man-made scale does permit them to have one thousand times as much income. In other words, it is much more difficult for a wealthy minority to affect a nation's U5MR, and it therefore presents a more accurate, if far from perfect, picture of the health status of the majority of children (and of society as a whole).

For these reasons, the U5MR is chosen by UNICEF as its single most important indicator of the state of a nation's children. That is why the statistical annex lists the nations of the world not in ascending order of their per capita GNP but in descending order of their under-five mortality rates.

The speed of progress in reducing the U5MR can be measured by calculating its average annual reduction rate (AARR). Unlike the comparison of absolute changes, the AARR reflects the fact that the lower limits to U5MR are approached only with increasing difficulty. As lower levels of under-five mortality are reached, for example, the same absolute reduction obviously represents a greater percentage of reduction. The AARR therefore shows a higher rate of progress for, say, a 10 point reduction if that reduction happens at a lower level of under-five mortality. (A fall in U5MR of 10 points from 100 to 90 represents a reduction of 10%, whereas the same 10-point fall from 20 to 10 represents a reduction of 50%.)

When used in conjunction with GNP growth rates, the U5MR and its reduction rate can therefore give a picture of the progress being made by any country or region, and over any period of time, towards the satisfaction of some of the most essential of human needs.

As table 9 shows, there is no fixed relationship between the annual reduction rate of the U5MR and the annual rate of growth in per capita GNP. Such comparisons help to throw the emphasis on to the policies, priorities, and other factors which determine the ratio between economic and social progress.

Finally, the table gives the total fertility rate for each country and its average annual rate of reduction. It will be seen that many of the nations which have achieved significant reductions in their U5MR have also achieved significant reductions in fertility.

Table 9: The rate of progress

		Under-5 mortality rate			average annual rate of reduction (%)			GNP per capita average annual growth rate (%)		Total fertility rate			average annual rate of reduction (%)	
		1960	1980	1992	1960-80	1980-92	required** 1992-2000	1965-80	1980-91	1960	1980	1992	1960-80	1980-92
1	Niger	320	320	320	0.0	0.0	19.0	-2.5	-4.1	7.1	7.1	7.1	0.0	0.0
2	Angola	345	261	292	1.4	-0.9	17.9	. .	6.1x	6.4	6.9	7.2	-0.4	-0.4
3	Mozambique	331	269	287	1.0	-0.5	17.6	. .	-1.1	6.3	6.5	6.5	-0.2	0.0
4	Afghanistan	360	280	257	1.3	0.7	16.3	0.6	. .	6.9	7.1	6.9	-0.1	0.2
5	Sierra Leone	385	301	249	1.2	1.6	15.9	0.7	-1.6	6.2	6.5	6.5	-0.2	0.0
6	Guinea-Bissau	336	290	239	0.7	1.6	15.3	-2.7	1.1	5.1	5.7	5.8	-0.6	-0.1
7	Guinea	337	276	230	1.0	1.5	14.9	1.3	. .	7.0	7.0	7.0	0.0	0.0
8	Malawi	365	290	226	1.1	2.1	14.6	3.2	0.1	6.9	7.6	7.6	-0.5	0.0
9	Rwanda	191	222	222	-0.8	0.0	14.4	1.6	-2.4	7.5	8.5	8.5	-0.6	0.0
10	Mali	400	310	220	1.3	2.9	14.3	2.1x	-0.1	7.1	7.1	7.1	0.0	0.0
11	Liberia	288	235	217	1.0	0.7	14.1	0.5	5.2x	6.6	6.8	6.8	-0.1	0.0
12	Somalia	294	246	211	0.9	1.3	13.8	-0.1	-1.8x	7.0	7.0	7.0	0.0	0.0
13	Chad	325	254	209	1.2	1.6	13.7	-1.9	3.8	6.0	5.9	5.9	0.1	0.0
14	Eritrea	294	260	208	0.6	1.9	13.6	. .	. .			5.8	. .	. .
15	Ethiopia	294	260	208	0.6	1.9	13.6	0.4	-1.6	6.7	6.8	7.0	-0.1	-0.2
16	Mauritania	321	249	206	1.3	1.6	13.5	-0.1	-1.8	6.5	6.5	6.5	0.0	0.0
17	Zambia	220	160	202	1.6	-1.9	13.2	-1.2	-2.9x	6.6	7.1	6.4	-0.4	0.9
18	Bhutan	324	249	201	1.3	1.8	13.2	. .	6.8	6.0	5.9	5.9	0.1	0.0
19	Nigeria	204	196	191	0.2	0.2	12.5	4.2	-2.3	6.8	6.9	6.5	-0.1	0.5
20	Zaire	286	204	188	1.7	0.7	12.3	-1.3	-1.6	6.0	6.6	6.7	-0.5	-0.1
21	Uganda	218	181	185	0.9	-0.2	12.1	-2.2	3.3	6.9	7.0	7.3	-0.1	-0.3
22	Cambodia	217	330	184	-2.1	4.9	12.1	. .	. .	6.3	4.5	4.5	1.7	0.0
23	Burundi	255	193	179	1.4	0.6	11.7	2.4	1.3	6.8	6.8	6.8	0.0	0.0
24	Central African Rep.	294	202	179	1.9	1.0	11.7	0.8	-1.4	5.6	6.0	6.2	-0.3	-0.3
25	Yemen	378	236	177	2.4	2.4	11.6	. .	. .	7.5	7.7	7.2	-0.1	0.6
26	Tanzania, U. Rep. of	249	202	176	1.0	1.2	11.5	0.8	-0.8	6.8	6.8	6.8	0.0	0.0
27	Ghana	215	157	170	1.6	-0.7	11.1	-0.8	-0.3	6.9	6.5	6.0	0.3	0.7
28	Madagascar	364	216	168	2.6	2.1	11.0	-0.4	-2.5	6.6	6.6	6.6	0.0	0.0
29	Sudan	292	210	166	1.7	2.0	10.8	0.8	-2.4	6.7	6.6	6.1	0.1	0.7
30	Gabon	287	194	158	2.0	1.7	10.1	5.6	-4.2	4.1	4.4	5.3	-0.4	-1.6
31	Lesotho	204	173	156	0.8	0.8	10.0	6.8	-0.5	5.8	5.6	4.7	0.2	1.5
32	Burkina Faso	318	218	150	1.9	3.1	9.5	1.7	1.2	6.4	6.5	6.5	-0.1	0.0
33	Benin	310	176	147	2.8	1.5	9.3	-0.3	-0.9	6.9	7.1	7.1	-0.1	0.0
34	Senegal	303	221	145	1.6	3.5	9.1	-0.5	0.1	7.0	6.9	6.1	0.1	1.0
35	Lao Peo. Dem. Rep.	233	190	145	1.0	2.3	9.1	. .	1.2	6.2	6.7	6.7	-0.4	0.0
36	Pakistan	221	151	137	1.9	0.8	8.4	1.8	3.2	6.9	7.0	6.2	-0.1	1.0
37	Togo	264	175	137	2.0	2.0	8.4	1.7	-1.3	6.6	6.6	6.6	0.0	0.0
38	Haiti	270	195	133	1.6	3.2	8.1	0.9	-2.4	6.3	5.3	4.8	0.9	0.8
39	Nepal	279	177	128	2.3	2.7	7.5	. .	2.1	5.8	6.4	5.5	-0.5	1.3
40	Bangladesh	247	211	127	0.8	4.2	7.4	-0.3	1.9	6.7	6.4	4.8	0.2	2.4
41	Côte d'Ivoire	300	180	124	2.6	3.1	7.1	2.8	-4.6	7.2	7.4	7.4	-0.1	0.0
42	India	236	177	124	1.4	3.0	7.1	1.5	3.2	5.9	4.8	3.9	1.0	1.7
43	Bolivia	252	170	118	2.0	3.0	6.5	1.7	-2.0	6.7	5.8	4.6	0.7	1.9
44	Cameroon	264	173	117	2.1	3.3	6.4	2.4	-1.0	5.8	6.4	5.7	-0.5	1.0
45	Myanmar	237	146	113	2.4	2.1	6.0	1.6	. .	6.0	5.1	4.2	0.8	1.6
46	Indonesia	216	128	111	2.6	1.2	5.8	5.2	3.9	5.5	4.4	3.1	1.1	2.9
47	Congo	220	125	110	2.8	1.1	5.6	2.7	-0.2	5.9	6.3	6.3	-0.3	0.0
48	Libyan Arab Jamahiriya	269	150	104	2.9	3.0	4.9	0.0	-9.2x	7.1	7.3	6.4	-0.1	1.1
49	Turkmenistan			91	. .	. .	. .	. .	0.7			4.5	. .	. .
50	Turkey	217	141	87	2.2	4.0	4.0	3.6	2.9	6.3	4.3	3.5	1.9	1.7
51	Zimbabwe	181	125	86	1.8	3.2	4.4	1.7	-0.2	7.5	6.4	5.4	0.8	1.4
52	Tajikistan	. .	. .	85	. .	. .	. .	. .	-0.1	. .	. .	5.3	. .	. .
53	Iraq	171	83	80	3.6	0.3	11.5	. .	. .	7.2	6.5	5.7	0.5	1.1
54	Mongolia	185	112	80	2.5	2.8	4.4	. .	. .	6.0	5.4	4.7	0.5	1.2
55	Namibia	206	114	79	3.0	3.1	4.4	. .	-1.2	6.0	6.0	6.0	0.0	0.0
56	Papua New Guinea	248	95	77	4.8	1.8	4.6	. .	-0.6	6.3	5.7	4.9	0.5	1.3
57	Guatemala	205	136	76	2.0	4.8	3.7	3.0	-1.8	6.9	6.3	5.4	0.5	1.3
58	Nicaragua	209	143	76	1.9	5.3	3.4	-0.7	-4.4	7.4	6.2	5.1	0.9	1.6
59	Kenya	202	112	74	2.9	3.5	4.4	3.1	0.3	8.0	7.8	6.3	0.1	1.8
60	Algeria	243	145	72	2.6	5.8	3.9	4.2	-0.7	7.3	6.8	4.9	0.4	2.7
61	South Africa	126	91	70	1.6	2.2	4.6	3.2	0.7	6.5	4.9	4.1	1.4	1.5
62	Uzbekistan	. .	. .	68	. .	. .	. .	. .	0.8	. .	. .	4.3	. .	. .
63	Brazil	181	93	65	3.3	2.9	4.3	6.3	0.5	6.2	4.0	2.8	2.2	3.0
64	Peru	236	130	65	3.0	5.8	3.5	0.8	-2.4	6.9	5.0	3.6	1.6	2.7
65	El Salvador	210	120	63	2.8	5.4	3.7	1.5	-0.3	6.8	5.4	4.1	1.2	2.3
66	Morocco	215	145	61	2.0	7.2	3.0	2.7	1.6	7.2	5.7	4.4	1.2	2.2
67	Kyrgyzstan	. .	. .	60	. .	. .	. .	. .	2.1	. .	. .	3.9	. .	. .
68	Philippines	102	70	60	1.9	1.2	4.7	3.2	-1.2	6.9	4.9	4.0	1.7	1.7
69	Ecuador	180	101	59	2.9	4.5	4.2	5.4	-0.6	6.9	5.1	3.7	1.5	2.7
70	Botswana	170	94	58	3.0	4.0	4.2	9.9	5.6	6.8	6.8	5.1	0.0	2.4
71	Honduras	203	100	58	3.6	4.5	4.2	1.1	-0.5	7.3	6.4	5.0	0.7	2.1
72	Iran, Islamic Rep. of	233	126	58	3.1	6.5	3.3	2.9	-1.3	7.2	6.5	6.0	0.5	0.7
73	Egypt	258	180	55	1.8	9.9	2.0	2.8	1.9	7.0	5.2	4.2	1.5	1.8
74	Azerbaijan	. .	. .	53	. .	. .	. .	. .	0.4	. .	. .	3.2	. .	. .
75	Dominican Rep.	152	94	50	2.4	5.2	3.6	3.8	-0.2	7.4	4.5	3.4	2.5	2.3

		Under-5 mortality rate			average annual rate of reduction (%)			GNP per capita average annual growth rate (%)		Total fertility rate			average annual rate of reduction (%)	
		1960	1980	1992	1960-80	1980-92	required** 1992-2000	1965-80	1980-91	1960	1980	1992	1960-80	1980-92
76	Kazakhstan	..	..	50	..	..	..	..	0.9	..	..	2.7	..	..
77	Viet Nam	219	105	49	3.7	6.3	3.7	..	..	6.0	5.1	3.9	0.8	2.2
78	Lebanon	91	62	44	1.9	2.8	4.2	..	..	6.3	4.0	3.1	2.3	2.1
79	China	209	65	43	5.9	3.4	5.1	4.1	7.8	5.7	2.7	2.2	3.7	1.7
80	Saudi Arabia	292	90	40	5.9	6.7	3.7	4.0x	-3.4	7.2	7.3	6.4	-0.1	1.1
81	Syrian Arab Rep.	201	73	40	5.1	5.0	3.8	5.1	-1.4	7.3	7.4	6.2	-0.1	1.5
82	Tunisia	244	102	38	4.4	8.2	2.7	4.7	1.1	7.1	5.3	3.5	1.5	3.5
83	Moldova	..	..	36	..	..	..	..	1.8	..	..	2.5	..	..
84	Albania	151	57	34	4.9	4.3	5.6	..	..	5.9	3.8	2.7	2.2	2.8
85	Armenia	..	..	34	..	..	..	..	2.1	..	..	3.0	..	..
86	Paraguay	90	61	34	1.9	4.9	4.0	4.1	-0.8	6.8	4.9	4.4	1.6	0.9
87	Korea, Dem. Peo. Rep.	120	43	33	5.1	2.3	4.4	..	..	5.8	3.1	2.4	3.1	2.1
88	Mexico	141	81	33	2.8	7.5	3.0	3.6	-0.5	6.8	4.7	3.2	1.8	3.2
89	Thailand	146	61	33	4.4	5.1	3.8	4.4	5.9	6.4	3.6	2.2	2.9	4.1
90	Russian Federation	..	..	32	..	..	..	..	1.3	..	..	1.8	..	..
91	Oman	300	95	31	5.7	9.3	3.6	9.0	4.4	7.2	7.2	6.8	0.0	0.5
92	Jordan	149	66	30	4.1	6.5	3.3	5.8x	-1.7	7.7	7.1	5.7	0.4	1.8
93	Georgia	..	..	29	..	..	..	..	2.2	..	..	2.1	..	..
94	Romania	82	36	28	4.1	2.0	3.0	..	0.0	2.3	2.4	2.1	-0.2	1.1
95	Latvia	..	..	26	..	..	..	..	2.8	1.9	2.0	2.0	-0.3	0.0
96	Ukraine	..	..	25	..	..	..	..	2.3	..	..	1.8	..	..
97	Argentina	68	41	24	2.5	4.5	4.1	1.7	-1.5	3.1	3.3	2.8	-0.3	1.4
98	Estonia	..	..	24	..	..	..	..	2.1	2.0	2.1	2.1	-0.2	0.0
99	Mauritius	84	42	24	3.4	4.7	4.2	3.7	6.1	5.9	2.8	2.0	3.7	2.8
100	Venezuela	70	42	24	2.6	4.6	4.1	2.3	-1.3	6.5	4.2	3.2	2.2	2.3
101	Belarus	..	..	23	..	..	..	..	3.3	..	..	1.9	..	..
102	Trinidad and Tobago	73	40	22	3.0	5.0	3.9	3.1	-5.2	5.2	3.3	2.8	2.3	1.4
103	United Arab Emirates	240	64	22	6.6	8.9	4.0	..	-5.8	6.9	5.4	4.5	1.2	1.5
104	Uruguay	47	42	22	0.6	5.3	4.3	2.5	-0.4	2.9	2.7	2.3	0.4	1.3
105	Yugoslavia (former)	113	37	22	5.6	4.4	4.5	5.2	-1.4	2.8	2.1	1.9	1.4	0.8
106	Colombia	132	59	20	4.1	8.9	4.4	3.7	1.2	6.8	3.8	2.7	2.9	2.8
107	Lithuania	..	..	20	..	..	..	..	2.5	2.5	2.1	2.0	0.9	0.4
108	Panama	104	31	20	6.0	3.7	4.5	2.8	-1.8	5.9	3.8	2.9	2.2	2.3
109	Bulgaria	70	25	20	5.1	1.9	6.3	..	1.7	2.2	2.1	1.8	0.2	1.3
110	Sri Lanka	130	52	19	4.6	8.4	2.7	2.8	2.5	5.3	3.5	2.5	2.1	2.8
111	Malaysia	105	42	19	4.6	6.6	4.0	4.7	2.9	6.8	4.2	3.7	2.4	1.1
112	Chile	138	35	18	6.9	5.5	3.6	0.0	1.6	5.3	2.8	2.7	3.2	0.3
113	Kuwait	128	35	17	6.6	6.1	5.2	0.6x	-2.2x	7.3	5.4	3.7	1.5	3.2
114	Poland	70	24	16	5.3	3.3	3.8	..	0.6	3.0	2.3	2.1	1.3	0.8
115	Hungary	57	26	16	3.9	4.0	4.9	5.1	0.7	2.0	2.0	1.8	0.0	0.9
116	Costa Rica	112	29	16	6.8	4.9	5.1	3.3	0.7	7.0	3.7	3.2	3.2	1.2
117	Jamaica	76	39	14	3.4	8.4	3.5	-0.1	0.0	5.4	3.8	2.4	1.8	3.8
118	Slovakia	..	..	14	..	..	..	..	..	..	..	2.0	..	..
119	Portugal	112	31	13	6.4	7.1	2.6	4.6	3.1	3.1	2.2	1.5	1.7	3.2
120	Czech Republic	..	..	12	..	..	..	..	..	..	..	1.9	..	..
121	Cuba	50	26	11	3.3	6.9	3.3	..	..	4.2	2.0	1.9	3.7	0.4
122	Israel	39	19	11	3.6	4.6	4.3	3.7	1.7	3.9	3.3	2.9	0.8	1.1
123	Belgium	35	15	11	4.3	2.8	6.5	3.6	2.0	2.6	1.7	1.6	2.1	0.5
124	USA	30	15	10	3.3	3.3	4.2	1.8	1.7	3.5	1.8	2.1	3.3	-1.3
125	New Zealand	26	16	10	2.5	3.7	2.3	1.7	0.7	3.9	2.1	2.1	3.1	0.0
126	Italy	50	17	10	5.3	4.9	4.9	3.2	2.2	2.4	1.7	1.3	1.7	2.2
127	Spain	57	16	9	6.2	4.5	5.0	4.1	2.8	2.8	2.2	1.4	1.2	3.8
128	Greece	64	23	9	5.2	7.5	2.9	4.8	1.1	2.2	2.1	1.5	0.2	2.8
129	Korea, Rep. of	124	18	9	9.8	5.3	3.7	7.3	8.7	5.7	2.6	1.7	3.9	3.5
130	Austria	43	17	9	4.6	5.5	4.2	4.0	2.1	2.7	1.6	1.5	2.6	0.5
131	France	34	13	9	4.9	3.0	4.6	3.7	1.8	2.8	1.9	1.8	1.9	0.5
132	United Kingdom	27	14	9	3.1	4.1	4.4	2.0	2.6	2.7	1.8	1.9	2.0	-0.5
133	Australia	24	13	9	3.0	3.8	3.7	2.2	1.6	3.3	2.0	1.9	2.5	0.5
134	Switzerland	27	11	9	4.5	2.1	4.1	1.5	1.6	2.4	1.5	1.6	2.4	-0.5
135	Germany	40	16	8	4.7	5.3	4.3	3.0x	2.2	2.4	1.5	1.5	2.4	0.0
136	Canada	33	13	8	4.8	3.7	4.5	3.3	2.0	3.8	1.7	1.8	4.0	-0.5
137	Denmark	25	10	8	4.4	2.3	3.3	2.2	2.2	2.6	1.6	1.7	2.4	-0.5
138	Norway	23	11	8	3.8	2.8	2.1	3.6	2.3	2.9	1.7	2.0	2.7	-1.4
139	Netherlands	22	11	7	3.4	3.2	3.3	2.7	1.6	3.1	1.5	1.7	3.6	-1.0
140	Sweden	20	9	7	4.1	1.6	6.0	2.0	1.7	2.3	1.6	2.1	1.8	-2.3
141	Hong Kong	52	13	7	6.9	5.2	4.5	6.2	5.6	5.0	2.1	1.4	4.3	3.4
142	Singapore	40	13	7	5.6	5.2	3.5	8.3	5.3	5.5	1.8	1.7	5.6	0.5
143	Finland	28	9	7	5.9	2.4	4.6	3.6	2.5	2.7	1.7	1.8	2.3	-0.5
144	Japan	40	11	6	6.6	4.5	5.0	5.1	3.6	2.0	1.8	1.7	0.5	0.5
145	Ireland	36	14	6	4.6	7.2	0.0	2.8	3.3	3.8	3.2	2.1	0.9	3.5

** The average annual reduction rate required to achieve an under-five mortality rate in all countries of 70 per 1000 live births or of two thirds the 1990 rate, whichever is the less.
Countries listed in descending order of their 1992 under-five mortality rates (table 1).

Table 10: Regional summaries

	Sub-Saharan Africa	Middle East and North Africa	South Asia	East Asia and Pacific	Latin America and Caribbean	Former USSR	Industrialized countries	Developing countries	Least developed countries
Table 1: Basic indicators									
Under-5 mortality rate 1960	255	240	237	200	157	. .	43	216	282
Under-5 mortality rate 1992	181	78	129	56	50	44	11	104	179
Infant mortality rate 1960	152	155	145	132	105	. .	36	137	171
Infant mortality rate 1992	111	57	88	42	39	36	9	70	114
Total population (millions)	533	341	1183	1728	451	292	936	4234	537
Annual no. of births (thousands)	24444	12087	37885	39550	11699	4705	12646	125665	23795
Annual no. of under-5 deaths (thousands)	4431	943	4884	2216	581	205	135	13056	4260
GNP per capita (US$)	505	1944	325	692	2345	2691	18884	843	240
Life expectancy at birth (years)	51	64	58	68	68	69	76	61	50
Total adult literacy rate (%)	51	58	46	76	85	. .	95	. .	43
% enrolled in primary school	68	95	86	125	107	. .	103	100	68
% share of household income, lowest 40%	. .	. .	21	18	10	. .	18	. .	. .
% share of household income, highest 20%	. .	. .	41	44	61	. .	40	. .	. .
Table 2: Nutrition									
% with low birth weight	16	10	34	11	11	. .	6	19	24
% of children who are exclusively breastfed, 0-3 months	26	. .	. .	. .	. .	. .	. .	. .	. .
% of children who are breastfed with food, 6-9 months	64	. .	. .	. .	. .	. .	. .	. .	. .
% of children who are still breastfeeding, 20-23 months	. .	. .	. .	. .	. .	. .	. .	. .	. .
% of children suffering from underweight, moderate & severe	31	17	60	26	11	. .	. .	36	43
% of children suffering from underweight, severe	9	. .	25	. .	2	. .	. .	12	. .
% of children suffering from wasting, moderate & severe	12	8	19	. .	4	. .	. .	10	17
% of children suffering from stunting, moderate & severe	49	31	64	. .	23	. .	. .	48	56
Total goitre rate (%)	16	23	13	13	15	. .	. .	15	20
Calorie supply as % of requirements	93	124	99	112	114	. .	134	107	90
% share of household consumption, all foods	38	39	51	45	34	. .	14	41	. .
% share of household consumption, cereals	15	10	19	. .	8	. .	2	. .	. .
Table 3: Health									
% with access to safe water, total	43	77	80	68	78	. .	. .	70	49
% with access to safe water, urban	75	94	85	83	87	. .	. .	85	64
% with access to safe water, rural	35	61	78	63	55	. .	. .	64	46
% with access to adequate sanitation, total	35	68	19	71	66	. .	. .	51	33
% with access to adequate sanitation, urban	57	93	54	70	80	. .	. .	70	61
% with access to adequate sanitation, rural	27	46	6	70	33	. .	. .	41	26
% with access to health services, total	56	78	52	87	74	. .	. .	77	48
% with access to health services, urban	. .	. .	. .	. .	. .	. .	. .	. .	. .
% with access to health services, rural	. .	. .	. .	. .	. .	. .	. .	. .	. .
% of 1-year-olds immunized against TB	62	85	93	93	87	90	77	86	70
% of 1-year-olds immunized against DPT	45	82	83	91	76	77	80	78	52
% of 1-year-olds immunized against polio	45	82	83	92	76	79	85	78	51
% of 1-year-olds immunized against measles	46	79	79	91	84	84	79	77	51
% of pregnant women immunized against tetanus	27	51	72	19	31	. .	. .	38	41
ORT use rate (%)	57	50	35	29	57	. .	. .	40	37
Table 4: Education									
Adult literacy rate 1970, male (%)	34	47	44	76	76	. .	97	53	36
Adult literacy rate 1970, female (%)	17	19	19	56	69	. .	95	33	18
Adult literacy rate 1990, male (%)	61	70	59	86	87	. .	. .	75	54
Adult literacy rate 1990, female (%)	41	46	32	67	83	. .	. .	55	32
No. of radio sets per 1000 population	147	248	77	197	338	. .	1166	177	97
No. of television sets per 1000 population	23	113	27	44	165	. .	549	55	9
Primary school enrolment ratio (%) 1960 (gross), male	46	72	77	120	75	. .	109	93	48
Primary school enrolment ratio (%) 1960 (gross), female	24	40	39	85	71	. .	107	62	23
Primary school enrolment ratio (%) 1986-91 (gross), male	76	103	97	128	105	. .	103	107	74
Primary school enrolment ratio (%) 1986-91 (gross), female	60	87	73	120	102	. .	103	92	57
Primary school enrolment ratio (%) 1986-91 (net), male	54	90	. .	. .	74	. .	97	87	55
Primary school enrolment ratio (%) 1986-91 (net), female	46	79	. .	. .	75	. .	97	82	45
% reaching final grade, primary school	58	85	53	79	48	. .	94	66	54
Secondary school enrolment ratio, male (%)	21	62	47	52	44	. .	91	47	21
Secondary school enrolment ratio, female (%)	14	45	28	43	48	. .	92	36	12

	Sub-Saharan Africa	Middle East and North Africa	South Asia	East Asia and Pacific	Latin America and Caribbean	Former USSR	Industrialized countries	Developing countries	Least developed countries
Table 5: Demographic indicators									
Population under 16 (millions)	258	149	464	542	167	80	200	1580	249
Population under 5 (millions)	100	54	161	185	55	26	62	554	95
Population annual growth rate 1965-80 (%)	2.8	2.8	2.3	2.2	2.5	. .	0.8	2.4	2.6
Population annual growth rate 1980-92 (%)	3.0	3.0	2.2	1.7	2.1	. .	0.6	2.1	2.7
Crude death rate 1960	24	21	21	19	13	. .	10	20	25
Crude death rate 1992	15	8	11	7	7	11	9	9	16
Crude birth rate 1960	49	47	44	39	42	. .	20	42	48
Crude birth rate 1992	45	35	32	23	26	16	14	30	44
Life expectancy 1960 (years)	40	47	43	47	56	. .	69	46	39
Life expectancy 1992 (years)	51	64	58	68	68	69	76	61	50
Total fertility rate	6.4	5.0	4.3	2.5	3.1	2.0	1.8	3.7	6.0
% of population urbanized	30	54	25	30	73	66	75	35	21
Urban population annual growth rate 1965-80 (%)	5.4	4.6	3.8	3.3	3.8	. .	1.4	3.9	5.5
Urban population annual growth rate 1980-92 (%)	5.1	4.6	3.5	4.1	3.0	. .	0.9	3.9	5.2
Table 6: Economic indicators									
GNP per capita (US$)	505	1944	325	692	2345	2691	18884	843	240
GNP per capita annual growth rate 1965-80 (%)	3.0	3.2	1.5	4.8	4.1	. .	2.9	3.7	0.4
GNP per capita annual growth rate 1980-91 (%)	-0.4	-0.7	3.1	6.6	-0.2	1.5	2.2	2.4	0.3
Annual rate of inflation (%)	15	14	8	6	211	. .	5	69	16
% below absolute poverty level, urban	. .	. .	33	. .	18	. .	. .	27	55
% below absolute poverty level, rural	62	. .	39	17	49	. .	. .	31	70
% of government expenditure to health	4	5	2	3	6	. .	13	4	5
% of government expenditure to education	12	18	3	16	9	. .	4	11	13
% of government expenditure to defence	9	15	18	13	5	. .	13	11	13
ODA inflow (US$ millions)	14548	10586	6612	7422	4283	. .	. .	43451	14263
ODA inflow as % of recipient GNP	10	2	2	1	0	. .	. .	1	15
Debt service, % of goods & services exports 1970	5	. .	21	. .	14	. .	. .	12	7
Debt service, % of goods & services exports 1991	16	28	24	11	22	. .	. .	18	12
Table 7: Women									
Life expectancy, females as % of males	107	104	101	106	109	. .	109	105	104
Adult literacy, females as % of males	68	66	54	78	96	. .	. .	74	58
Enrolment, females as % of males, primary school	80	84	75	93	98	. .	100	87	78
Enrolment, females as % of males, secondary school	66	72	60	82	109	. .	102	77	58
Contraceptive prevalence (%)	12	39	38	73	59	. .	71	53	13
Pregnant women immunized against tetanus (%)	27	51	72	19	31	. .	. .	38	41
% of births attended by trained health personnel	37	56	29	81	81	. .	98	55	28
Maternal mortality rate	610	200	490	160	180	. .	10	350	590
Table 9: The rate of progress									
Under-5 mortality rate 1960	255	240	237	200	157	. .	43	216	282
Under-5 mortality rate 1980	203	144	179	80	86	. .	17	138	222
Under-5 mortality rate 1992	181	78	129	56	50	44	11	104	179
Under-5 mortality annual reduction rate 1960-80 (%)	1.2	2.5	1.4	4.6	3.0	. .	4.6	2.2	1.2
Under-5 mortality annual reduction rate 1980-92 (%)	0.9	5.1	2.7	3.0	4.6	. .	3.9	2.4	1.8
Under-5 mortality annual reduction rate required 1992-2000 (%)	12.3	5.8	7.7	5.1	4.2	. .	4.3	7.9	11.8
GNP per capita annual growth rate 1965-80 (%)	3.0	3.2	1.5	4.8	4.1	. .	2.9	3.7	0.4
GNP per capita annual growth rate 1980-91 (%)	-0.4	-0.7	3.1	6.6	-0.2	1.5	2.2	2.4	0.3
Total fertility rate 1960	6.7	7.0	6.1	5.8	6.0	. .	2.8	6.0	6.5
Total fertility rate 1980	6.7	5.9	5.2	3.2	4.2	. .	1.9	4.4	6.5
Total fertility rate 1992	6.4	5.0	4.3	2.5	3.1	2.0	1.8	3.7	6.0
Total fertility annual reduction rate 1960-80 (%)	0.0	0.9	0.8	3.0	1.8	. .	1.9	1.6	0.0
Total fertility annual reduction rate 1980-92 (%)	0.4	1.4	1.6	2.1	2.5	. .	0.5	1.4	0.7

Figures in this table are totals or weighted averages.

COUNTRY
GROUPINGS

SUB-SAHARAN AFRICA

Angola	Eritrea	Malawi	Sierra Leone
Benin	Ethiopia	Mali	Somalia
Botswana	Gabon	Mauritania	South Africa
Burkina Faso	Ghana	Mauritius	Tanzania, U. Rep. of
Burundi	Guinea	Mozambique	Togo
Cameroon	Guinea-Bissau	Namibia	Uganda
Central African Rep.	Kenya	Niger	Zaire
Chad	Lesotho	Nigeria	Zambia
Congo	Liberia	Rwanda	Zimbabwe
Côte d'Ivoire	Madagascar	Senegal	

MIDDLE EAST AND NORTH AFRICA

Algeria	Kuwait	Saudi Arabia	United Arab Emirates
Egypt	Lebanon	Sudan	Yemen
Iran, Islamic Rep. of	Libyan Arab Jamahiriya	Syrian Arab Rep.	
Iraq	Morocco	Tunisia	
Jordan	Oman	Turkey	

SOUTH ASIA

Afghanistan	Bhutan	Nepal	Sri Lanka
Bangladesh	India	Pakistan	

EAST ASIA AND PACIFIC

Cambodia	Korea, Dem. Peo. Rep.	Mongolia	Singapore
China	Korea, Rep. of	Myanmar	Thailand
Hong Kong	Lao Peo. Dem. Rep.	Papua New Guinea	Viet Nam
Indonesia	Malaysia	Philippines	

LATIN AMERICA AND CARIBBEAN

Argentina	Cuba	Honduras	Peru
Bolivia	Dominican Rep.	Jamaica	Trinidad and Tobago
Brazil	Ecuador	Mexico	Uruguay
Chile	El Salvador	Nicaragua	Venezuela
Colombia	Guatemala	Panama	
Costa Rica	Haiti	Paraguay	

FORMER USSR

Armenia	Georgia	Lithuania	Turkmenistan
Azerbaijan	Kazakhstan	Moldova	Ukraine
Belarus	Kyrgyzstan	Russian Federation	Uzbekistan
Estonia	Latvia	Tajikistan	

INDUSTRIALIZED COUNTRIES

Albania	Finland	Japan	Spain
Australia	France	Netherlands	Sweden
Austria	Germany	New Zealand	Switzerland
Belgium	Greece	Norway	United Kingdom
Bulgaria	Hungary	Poland	USA
Canada	Ireland	Portugal	Yugoslavia (former)
Czech Republic	Israel	Romania	
Denmark	Italy	Slovakia	

DEVELOPING COUNTRIES

Afghanistan	Egypt	Liberia	Rwanda
Algeria	El Salvador	Libyan Arab Jamahiriya	Saudi Arabia
Angola	Eritrea	Madagascar	Senegal
Argentina	Ethiopia	Malawi	Sierra Leone
Bangladesh	Gabon	Malaysia	Singapore
Benin	Ghana	Mali	Somalia
Bhutan	Guatemala	Mauritania	South Africa
Bolivia	Guinea	Mauritius	Sri Lanka
Botswana	Guinea-Bissau	Mexico	Sudan
Brazil	Haiti	Mongolia	Syrian Arab Rep.
Burkina Faso	Honduras	Morocco	Tanzania, U. Rep. of
Burundi	Hong Kong	Mozambique	Thailand
Cambodia	India	Myanmar	Togo
Cameroon	Indonesia	Namibia	Trinidad and Tobago
Central African Rep.	Iran, Islamic Rep. of	Nepal	Tunisia
Chad	Iraq	Nicaragua	Turkey
Chile	Jamaica	Niger	Uganda
China	Jordan	Nigeria	United Arab Emirates
Colombia	Kenya	Oman	Uruguay
Congo	Korea, Dem. Peo. Rep.	Pakistan	Venezuela
Costa Rica	Korea, Rep. of	Panama	Viet Nam
Côte d'Ivoire	Kuwait	Papua New Guinea	Yemen
Cuba	Lao Peo. Dem. Rep.	Paraguay	Zaire
Dominican Rep.	Lebanon	Peru	Zambia
Ecuador	Lesotho	Philippines	Zimbabwe

LEAST DEVELOPED COUNTRIES

Afghanistan	Chad	Malawi	Somalia
Bangladesh	Ethiopia	Mali	Sudan
Benin	Guinea	Mauritania	Tanzania, U. Rep. of
Bhutan	Guinea-Bissau	Mozambique	Togo
Botswana	Haiti	Myanmar	Uganda
Burkina Faso	Lao Peo. Dem. Rep.	Nepal	Yemen
Burundi	Lesotho	Niger	Zaire
Cambodia	Liberia	Rwanda	Zambia
Central African Rep.	Madagascar	Sierra Leone	

DEFINITIONS

Under-five mortality rate

Number of deaths of children under five years of age per 1,000 live births. More specifically this is the probability of dying between birth and exactly five years of age.

Infant mortality rate

Number of deaths of infants under one year of age per 1,000 live births. More specifically this is the probability of dying between birth and exactly one year of age.

GNP

Gross national product, expressed in current United States dollars. GNP per capita growth rates are average annual growth rates that have been computed by fitting trend lines to the logarithmic values of GNP per capita at constant market prices for each year of the time period.

Life expectancy at birth

The number of years newborn children would live if subject to the mortality risks prevailing for the cross-section of population at the time of their birth.

Adult literacy rate

Percentage of persons aged 15 and over who can read and write.

Primary and secondary enrolment ratios

The gross enrolment ratio is the total number of children enrolled in a schooling level – whether or not they belong in the relevant age group for that level – expressed as a percentage of the total number of children in the relevant age group for that level. The net enrolment ratio is the total number of children enrolled in a schooling level who belong in the relevant age group, expressed as a percentage of the total number in that age group.

Income share

Percentage of private income received by the highest 20% and lowest 40% of households.

Low birth weight

Less than 2,500 grammes.

Underweight

Moderate and severe – below minus two standard deviations from median weight for age of reference population;
severe – below minus three standard deviations from median weight for age of reference population.

Wasting

Moderate and severe – below minus two standard deviations from median weight for height of reference population.

Stunting

Moderate and severe – below minus two standard deviations from median height for age of reference population.

Total goitre rate

Percentage of children aged 6-11 with palpable or visible goitre. This is an indicator of iodine deficiency, which causes brain damage and mental retardation.

Access to health services

Percentage of the population that can reach appropriate local health services by the local means of transport in no more than one hour.

DPT

Diphtheria, pertussis (whooping cough) and tetanus.

ORT use

Percentage of all cases of diarrhoea in children under five years of age treated with oral rehydration salts or an appropriate household solution.

Children reaching final grade of primary school

Percentage of the children entering the first grade of primary school who eventually reach the final grade.

Crude death rate

Annual number of deaths per 1,000 population.

Crude birth rate

Annual number of births per 1,000 population.

Total fertility rate

The number of children that would be born per woman, if she were to live to the end of her child-bearing years and bear children at each age in accordance with prevailing age-specific fertility rates.

Urban population

Percentage of population living in urban areas as defined according to the national definition used in the most recent population census.

Absolute poverty level

The income level below which a minimum nutritionally adequate diet plus essential non-food requirements is not affordable.

ODA

Official development assistance.

Debt service

The sum of interest payments and repayments of principal on external public and publicly guaranteed long-term debts.

Contraceptive prevalence

Percentage of married women aged 15-49 currently using contraception.

Births attended

Percentage of births attended by physicians, nurses, midwives, trained primary health care workers or trained traditional birth attendants.

Maternal mortality rate

Number of deaths of women from pregnancy related causes per 100,000 live births.

MAIN SOURCES

Under-five and infant mortality

United Nations Population Division, UNICEF, United Nations Statistical Division, World Bank and US Bureau of the Census.

Total population

United Nations Population Division.

Births

United Nations Population Division, United Nations Statistical Division and World Bank.

Under-five deaths

United Nations Population Division and UNICEF.

GNP per capita

World Bank.

Life expectancy

United Nations Population Division.

Adult literacy

United Nations Educational, Scientific and Cultural Organization (UNESCO).

School enrolment and completion

United Nations Educational, Scientific and Cultural Organization (UNESCO).

Household income

World Bank.

Low birth weight

World Health Organization (WHO).

Breastfeeding

Demographic and Health Surveys, (Institute for Resource Development), and World Health Organization (WHO).

Underweight, wasting and stunting

World Health Organization (WHO) and Demographic and Health Surveys.

Goitre rate

World Health Organization (WHO).

Calorie intake

Food and Agriculture Organization of the United Nations (FAO).

Household expenditure on food

World Bank.

Access to drinking water and sanitation facilities

World Health Organization (WHO) and UNICEF.

Access to health services

UNICEF.

Immunization

World Health Organization (WHO) and UNICEF.

ORT use

World Health Organization (WHO).

Radio and television

United Nations Educational, Scientific and Cultural Organization (UNESCO).

Child population

United Nations Population Division.

Crude death and birth rates

United Nations Population Division.

Fertility

United Nations Population Division.

Urban population

United Nations Population Division and World Bank

Inflation and absolute poverty level

World Bank.

Expenditure on health, education and defence

World Bank and International Monetary Fund (IMF).

ODA

Organisation for Economic Co-operation and Development (OECD).

Debt service

World Bank.

Contraceptive prevalence

United Nations Population Division, Rockefeller Foundation and Demographic and Health Surveys.

Births attended

World Health Organization (WHO).

Maternal mortality

World Health Organization (WHO).

UNICEF Headquarters
UNICEF House, 3 UN Plaza, New York,
NY 10017, USA

UNICEF Geneva Office
Palais des Nations, CH-1211 Geneva 10,
Switzerland

UNICEF Regional Office for Eastern and
Southern Africa
P.O. Box 44145, Nairobi, Kenya

UNICEF Regional Office for West and
Central Africa
P.O. Box 443, Abidjan 04, Côte d'Ivoire

UNICEF Regional Office for Latin America
and the Caribbean
Apartado Aéreo 7555, Santa Fé de Bogotá,
Colombia

UNICEF Regional Office for East Asia and
the Pacific
P.O. Box 2-154, Bangkok 10200, Thailand

UNICEF Regional Office for the Middle
East and North Africa
P.O. Box 811721, Amman, Jordan

UNICEF Regional Office for South Asia
P.O. Box 5815, Lekhnath Marg,
Kathmandu, Nepal

UNICEF Office for Australia and New
Zealand
P.O. Box Q143, Queen Victoria Building,
Sydney, N.S.W. 2000, Australia

UNICEF Office for Japan
Shin Aoyama Building Nishikan 22nd floor
1-1, Minami-Aoyama 1-Chome, Minato-ku,
Tokyo 107, Japan